NATIONAL ACADEMIES *Medicine*

Washington, DC

Aligning Investments in Therapeutic Development with Therapeutic Need

Closing the Gap

Donald Berwick, Ellen MacKenzie, Alex Helman, and Samantha Schumm, *Editors*

Committee on Strategies to Better Align Investments in Innovations for Therapeutic Development with Disease Burden and Unmet Needs

Board of Health Care Services

Health and Medicine Division

Consensus Study Report

NATIONAL ACADEMIES PRESS 500 Fifth Street, NW Washington, DC 20001

This activity was supported by contracts between the National Academy of Sciences and Gates Ventures and Peterson Center on Healthcare. Any opinions, findings, conclusions, or recommendations expressed in this publication do not necessarily reflect the views of any organization or agency that provided support for the project.

International Standard Book Number-10: 0-309-99382-1
Digital Object Identifier: https://doi.org/10.17226/29157
Library of Congress Control Number: 2025944626

This publication is available from the National Academies Press, 500 Fifth Street, NW, Keck 360, Washington, DC 20001; (800) 624-6242; https://nap. nationalacademies.org/.

The manufacturer's authorized representative in the European Union for product safety is Authorised Rep Compliance Ltd., Ground Floor, 71 Lower Baggot Street, Dublin D02 P593 Ireland; www.arccompliance.com.

Suggested citation: National Academies of Sciences, Engineering, and Medicine. 2025. *Aligning investments in therapeutic development with therapeutic need: Closing the gap.* Washington, DC: National Academies Press. https://doi. org/10.17226/29157.

The **National Academy of Sciences** was established in 1863 by an Act of Congress, signed by President Lincoln, as a private, nongovernmental institution to advise the nation on issues related to science and technology. Members are elected by their peers for outstanding contributions to research. Dr. Marcia McNutt is president.

The **National Academy of Engineering** was established in 1964 under the charter of the National Academy of Sciences to bring the practices of engineering to advising the nation. Members are elected by their peers for extraordinary contributions to engineering. Dr. Tsu-Jae Liu is president.

The **National Academy of Medicine** (formerly the Institute of Medicine) was established in 1970 under the charter of the National Academy of Sciences to advise the nation on medical and health issues. Members are elected by their peers for distinguished contributions to medicine and health. Dr. Victor J. Dzau is president.

The three Academies work together as the **National Academies of Sciences, Engineering, and Medicine** to provide independent, objective analysis and advice to the nation and conduct other activities to solve complex problems and inform public policy decisions. The National Academies also encourage education and research, recognize outstanding contributions to knowledge, and increase public understanding in matters of science, engineering, and medicine.

Learn more about the National Academies of Sciences, Engineering, and Medicine at **www.nationalacademies.org**.

COMMITTEE ON STRATEGIES TO BETTER ALIGN INVESTMENTS IN INNOVATIONS FOR THERAPEUTIC DEVELOPMENT WITH DISEASE BURDEN AND UNMET NEEDS

DONALD M. BERWICK (*Cochair*), Institute for Healthcare Improvement

ELLEN MacKENZIE (*Cochair*), Johns Hopkins University Bloomberg School of Public Health

STACEY J. ADAM, Foundation for the National Institutes of Health

MARIA ELENA BOTTAZZI, Baylor College of Medicine and Texas Children's Hospital

MACARIUS MWINISUNGEE DONNEYONG, The Ohio State University

STACIE B. DUSETZINA, Vanderbilt University School of Medicine

HOLLY FERNANDEZ LYNCH, University of Pennsylvania

TIMIAN M. GODFREY, University of Arizona College of Nursing (*until November 20, 2024*)

HOWARD SCOTT HOWELL, Blue Line Advisors, LLC; University of California, Berkeley; The Ohio State University

MARK OLFSON, Columbia University; New York State Psychiatric Institute

LISA LARRIMORE OUELLETTE, Stanford University

EDITH A. PEREZ, Mayo Clinic

KATHRYN A. PHILLIPS, University of California, San Francisco

JOSHUA A. SALOMON, Stanford University

DAVID I. SCHEER, Scheer & Company, Inc.; OrphAI Therapeutics, Inc.; Refactor Health; Adela, Inc.; and BiologicsMD, Inc.

WU ZENG, Georgetown University

Study Staff

ALEX HELMAN, Study Director and Senior Program Officer (*as of September 16, 2024*)

VERONICA WALLACE, Study Director and Senior Program Officer (*until September 16, 2024*)

SAMANTHA SCHUMM, Program Officer (*from September 30, 2024, to April 25, 2025*)

AJA DRAIN, Research Associate (*as of November 27, 2023*)

ANDREW MARCH, Program Officer (*as of April 16, 2025*)

ASHLEY BOLOGNA, Research Assistant (*as of October 18, 2024*)

ELIZA SOUSER, Senior Program Assistant (*from October 16, 2023, until August 23, 2024*)

RACHEL AMHAUS, Program Assistant (*from August 26, 2024, until October 17, 2024*)

Reviewers

This Consensus Study Report was reviewed in draft form by individuals chosen for their diverse perspectives and technical expertise. The purpose of this independent review is to provide candid and critical comments that will assist the National Academies of Sciences, Engineering, and Medicine in making each published report as sound as possible and to ensure that it meets the institutional standards for quality, objectivity, evidence, and responsiveness to the study charge. The review comments and draft manuscript remain confidential to protect the integrity of the deliberative process.

We thank the following individuals for their review of this report:

RODOLPHE BARRANGOU, North Carolina State University
BAINDU BAYON PAICELY, Saint Mary's College of California
A. MARK FENDRICK, University of Michigan
RICHARD FRANK, Brookings Institution
LAURA FRIEDEL, Tarplin, Downs & Young
BOB KOCKER, University of Southern California Schaeffer Center; Stanford Medicine; and Venrock
DEBRA G.B. LEONARD, University of Vermont
JOSEPH MILLUM, University of St. Andrews
ALI MOKDAD, University of Washington
JOHN E. NIEDERHUBER, Johns Hopkins University
RESHMA RAMACHANDRAN, Yale University
ANN E. TAYLOR, Comanche Biopharma; UnLearn AI; and the TB Alliance

DOUGLAS C. THROCKMORTON, Food and Drug Administration
  (*retired*)
KIMBERLEE TRZECIAK, Capitol Hill Consulting Group
SEAN TUNIS, Rubix Health; and Tufts Medical Center

Although the reviewers listed above provided many constructive comments and suggestions, they were not asked to endorse the conclusions or recommendations of this report, nor did they see the final draft before its release. The review of this report was overseen by **ALFRED BERG,** University of Washington, and **WALTER FRONTERA,** University of Puerto Rico. They were responsible for making certain that an independent examination of this report was carried out in accordance with the standards of the National Academies and that all review comments were carefully considered. Responsibility for the final content rests entirely with the authoring committee and the National Academies.

Acknowledgments

To begin, the committee would like to express its gratitude to the sponsors of this study. Funds for the committee's work were provided by Gates Ventures and the Peterson Center on Healthcare.

Numerous individuals and organizations made important contributions to the study process and this report by providing public testimony, submitting written comments, and more. The committee wishes to express its gratitude for each of these contributions, although space does not permit identifying them all here.

The committee wishes to express special thanks to Stephen Lim, professor and senior director at the Institute for Health Metrics and Evaluation, who served as a consultant to the committee and generously shared data to help the committee with its analysis on investments from industry. The committee would also like to thank the two National Academy of Medicine fellows, Drs. Sanket Dhruva and Inmaculada Hernandez, for their contributions throughout its work.

Lastly, the committee would like to express its gratitude to the National Academies' staff, who were critical in guiding their work. The committee gives a special thanks to Aja Drain for her research assistance and for being such a positive light throughout this committee process.

Contents

APPENDIXES

Preface

We can summarize the statement of task for our committee in four questions: (1) Given the current and future burdens of illness in the United States, what are the unmet needs for medications to treat them? (2) What medications are now, or will soon be, under development? (3) How well aligned, or mismatched, are the answers to Questions 1 and 2? (4) To the degree they are mismatched, why? And what changes in policy, payment, investment, and incentives would help close the gap?

Simple to ask, but hard to answer.

Question 1 calls for data on patterns of burden of illness that are accessible from a variety of sources, but "burden of disease" is multidimensional and eludes a consensus definition. Moreover, uncovering how to define "effectiveness" for the myriad of illnesses, and which needs are "unmet" proves to be a difficult task. Furthermore, assessing the degree of unmet needs turns out to require not just statistical and epidemiological analysis, but also value judgments when comparing the multiple dimensions of need across different conditions. For example, how shall rare but serious diseases be compared with more common ones through the lens of need? The committee eschewed a simple numerical comparison, but what, then, is the measuring stick?

Question 2 is even harder than Question 1, in part because the relevant information lies largely in the private sector, is largely proprietary, and is nowhere assembled into large, openly accessible databases that embrace both public and private sources. Moreover, what metric of "development" works well? The dollars in research budgets? The number of drugs trials? Patents issued?

Answering Question 3 (How big is the mismatch?) would require access to and aggregation of largely proprietary information on private-sector drug development, as well as difficult-to-estimate probabilities of success for medications now in the research pipeline. The Food and Drug Administration (FDA), foundations, and the private sector have a great deal of information on proposals for drug development and approval, but much of it was not accessible to us owing to its proprietary nature.

And Question 4, about achieving better alignment between unmet need and investment, surfaces how little we actually know about which policies and payments truly have leverage and which do not. Despite 4 decades of policy initiatives with the intent to encourage specific investments, including, for example, the 1983 Orphan Drug Act, priority review voucher programs, modifications in patent protections, and changes in FDA review and approval criteria, the landscape has much more opinion than hard evidence about their effect on decision making for investment, and the two—opinion and evidence—often conflict.

In spite of the challenges described above, our committee stepped cautiously and thoughtfully into this difficult terrain. As cochairs, we were fortunate to have a group of unusually expansive breadth in experience, subject-matter knowledge, and research experience. Among the members were clinicians; senior researchers; experts in law and ethics, drug development, market access, and investments; seasoned public servants; epidemiologists; and statisticians. Importantly, the committee also included members who had real or perceived conflicts of interests, but whose expertise was judged essential to our deliberations and who participated only with full transparency as to their roles and interests.[1] They proved invaluable to the process.

Our Consensus Report reflects more than a year of careful deliberations. Some uncertainties were resolved as we went along, such as our emerging, shared realization that no single metric of "burden" or "unmet need" would be feasible, as value judgments overlapped inevitably with evidence and data. We also developed a much better and more nuanced view of the historical role of FDA, and a view that, on the whole, to the degree that investments are not matching unmet needs, FDA, far from being a root cause of the gap, has been, to the extent law allows, a constructive and valuable force for improvement. Similarly, the National Institutes of Health (NIH) and its centers play a vital role in the pipeline of drug discovery. Indeed the investment of the United States in innovative research that saves lives and improves the public's health has, for many years, been revered around the world.

---

[1] See Appendix C for Disclosures of Unavoidable Conflicts of Interest.

However, at the time of release, the innovation ecosystem, federal funding, and institutional architecture are undergoing unprecedented and rapid change, seriously threatening our ability to sustain this position. Terminating grants midstream, as is currently being done, and limiting opportunities for new research that is judged important and scientifically sound by an independent community of peer scientists will likely impede innovation. The committee strongly recommends bipartisan congressional and executive branch support of NIH, FDA, and other federal agencies that are vital to the continued success of the biomedical research enterprise in the United States.

Other uncertainties proved more challenging, such as how to judge the widespread lack of evidence to support the effectiveness of currently available policy initiatives that purportedly aim to address unmet need whose supporters have strongly held views and important anecdotal testimony. More than once, we heard "absence of evidence is not evidence of absence" from those who believe strongly in the value of some of these initiatives, such as priority review vouchers or Orphan Drug Act subsidies. Our recommendations, we believe, reflect a prudent middle road.

As if the Statement of Task were not broad and challenging enough, our committee's mandate did not extend to addressing the root causes of a substantial portion of unmet need in America. Although access to existing therapeutic innovations, itself, was not a major focus of our Statement of Task, it would be naïve and harmful in the extreme in a report on unmet needs not to flag persistent inequities affecting access to treatment, as elevated in the fundamental National Academies report *Unequal Treatment: Confronting Racial and Ethnic Disparities in Health Care*, as a major reason for remediable disparities in health care and health in America.

The science is unequivocal and the implications unavoidable that racial, socioeconomic, and other forms of inequality in the United States affect and, in many cases, cause underinvestment in needed treatments and cures and, even more powerfully, create barriers to access and adherence to effective treatments, once developed.[2,3]

Any commitment to closing the gaps between unmet needs and therapy development must include a commitment to improving the policies and practices intended to eliminate or at least reduce existing disparities in access and use. Even the most efficacious drug therapy will miss meeting important proportions of unmet needs if not available and accessible to those most in need.

---

[2] National Academies of Sciences, Engineering, and Medicine. 2024. *Ending Unequal Treatment: Strategies to Achieve Equitable Health Care and Optimal Health for All*. Washington, DC: The National Academies Press. https://doi.org/10.17226/27820.

[3] Institute of Medicine. 2003. *Unequal Treatment: Confronting Racial and Ethnic Disparities in Health Care*. Washington, DC: The National Academies Press. https://doi.org/10.17226/12875.

We would like to express our deepest thanks to our committee members and the National Academy of Medicine Fellows who joined our deliberations. We have rarely experienced a group process endowed with such gracious listening and authentic dialogue among members who did not always agree at the start and whose convictions ran deep. That we arrived at a Consensus Report with which all now concur and that was not watered down testifies to this group's maturity and skills. Equally, we are all deeply in debt to the marvelous National Academies staff who supported our work and, in many ways, led us. There would have been no report without them.

> Donald Berwick and Ellen MacKenzie, *Cochairs*
> Committee on Strategies to Better Align Investments
> in Innovations for Therapeutic Development with
> Disease Burden and Unmet Needs
> May 2025

Summary[1]

The United States has long been a leader in biomedical research, generating new therapeutic breakthroughs and innovations that advance the health of our nation and the world. Research in both the public and private sectors contributes to the greater understanding of human health and disease and to the development of new technologies that lead to exciting clinical benefits for patients.

However, conducting this important research requires making complex decisions about where to focus resources and investment. In principle, investment in therapeutic development should follow the diseases and conditions with the highest unmet need and burden of disease. But both public and private funders developing therapeutics consider disease burden and unmet need in the context of myriad other competing considerations and goals in determining where to invest, such as limited funding; balancing advancements in basic, translational, and clinical science; advocacy from patient groups; the likelihood of regulatory approval and associated challenges; payer reimbursement; market competition; and overall timing and overall profits and return on investment. These competing practical and financial priorities do not always align with diseases with the highest burden and unmet needs. In addition, how to fairly allocate resources for drug development among potential beneficiaries involves ethical considerations and value judgments about which there is not universal agreement and for which there are a multitude of defensible approaches.

---

[1] References are not included in this report summary. Citations appear in subsequent report chapters. Key terms used in this summary and throughout the report are defined in Box 1-2.

These competing goals and judgments can hinder the research system's ability to prioritize disease burden and unmet need. For example, despite considerable investment in therapeutic development in the United States, substantial disease burden and unmet need remain in areas such as treatment for mental illness, cancer, cardiovascular disease, Alzheimer's disease, and immunological disorders to name a few, as well as broadly across the realm of rare and neglected tropical diseases. Some diseases and conditions have no available therapies, and often the existing, approved therapies are only modestly effective, have unclear clinical benefits, or have significant safety risks. Thus, the current system of drug development needs adjusting to improve the alignment of public and private investment in therapeutics with areas of unmet needs.

COMMITTEE TASK AND APPROACH

With support from Gates Ventures and the Peterson Center on Healthcare, the National Academies of Sciences, Engineering, and Medicine formed the Committee on Strategies to Better Align Investments in Innovations for Therapeutic Development with Disease Burden and Unmet Needs. The committee consisted of 16 members with a broad range of expertise, including health economics, data science, epidemiology, health policy, biomedical and pharmaceutical sciences, therapeutic development (including those with experience in the biopharmaceutical industry and the investment community), regulatory oversight, health law, bioethics, social, and behavioral sciences, clinical care, and health disparities. The committee was tasked with describing current U.S. disease burden, characterizing the degree and patterns of mismatch between that burden and public and private innovation in therapeutic development, describing challenges in better aligning innovations in therapeutic development with disease burden and unmet need, and proposing strategies and recommendations to improve alignment.

The committee approached its statement of task with the objective of designing policies such that society invests in innovation (including public and private investments) up to the point where the marginal cost equals the expected marginal social benefit of those investments. While cost is relatively straightforward to calculate (i.e., as the sum of private and public investment), the expected social benefit of these investments is complicated to determine. Benefit depends on the estimated reduction in disease burden for a given investment as well as on ethical judgments about how to value different kinds of health gains and inequality reductions, depending, for example, on such factors as the size of the population affected, disease severity in the context of duration or quality of life, the age of typically affected patients, and prevalence among otherwise marginalized groups. Therefore, rather than prescribing a single approach to calculating disease

burden and unmet need or providing a definitive list of disease or therapeutic areas where investments should be directed, the committee sought
to provide guidance that could accommodate different values and priorities
while still facilitating alignment among innovation, disease burden, and
unmet need. To demonstrate the barriers and solutions to misalignment,
the committee developed a conceptual framework that outlines key themes
of this report (Figure S-1).

The committee's recommendations are organized around five goals,
which are discussed in the following sections:

1. Design a state-of-the-art publicly accessible system to assess and
   track unmet need associated with U.S. disease burden, with a critical focus on identifying areas of mismatch and reducing health
   disparities.
2. Support and strengthen public investments in innovative therapeutics that address unmet need.
3. Strengthen public–private partnerships to encourage the sharing of
   information and technology transfer to facilitate addressing unmet
   need.
4. Strengthen a regulatory environment that supports innovation to
   address unmet need.
5. Strengthen a fiscal and policy environment to align reimbursement
   policy with evidence-based therapeutic value and the extent to
   which products address unmet need.

EVALUATING DISEASE BURDEN AND UNMET NEED

Although there is not a single metric universally accepted to measure
disease burden, unmet need, or innovation, the committee examined the
literature and spoke with outside experts to better understand the extent
to which there is a mismatch in investments for innovation with disease
burden and unmet need. The committee found that the current data on
U.S. disease burden, unmet need, and investment in therapeutic development have significant gaps and limitations. Although there are some existing data, they are not regularly compiled and synthesized for assessing
mismatch across factors. As a result of these limitations in the data, this
committee lacked the data needed to produce a comprehensive evaluation
of all aspects of disease burden, unmet need, and investment to fully assess
the mismatch. However, the committee did find that some therapeutic areas
are underinvested in relative to disease burden, such as chronic conditions
like cardiovascular disease and chronic obstructive pulmonary disease.
The committee's analysis of National Institutes of Health (NIH) funding
versus disease burden also highlighted the lower public investment in such

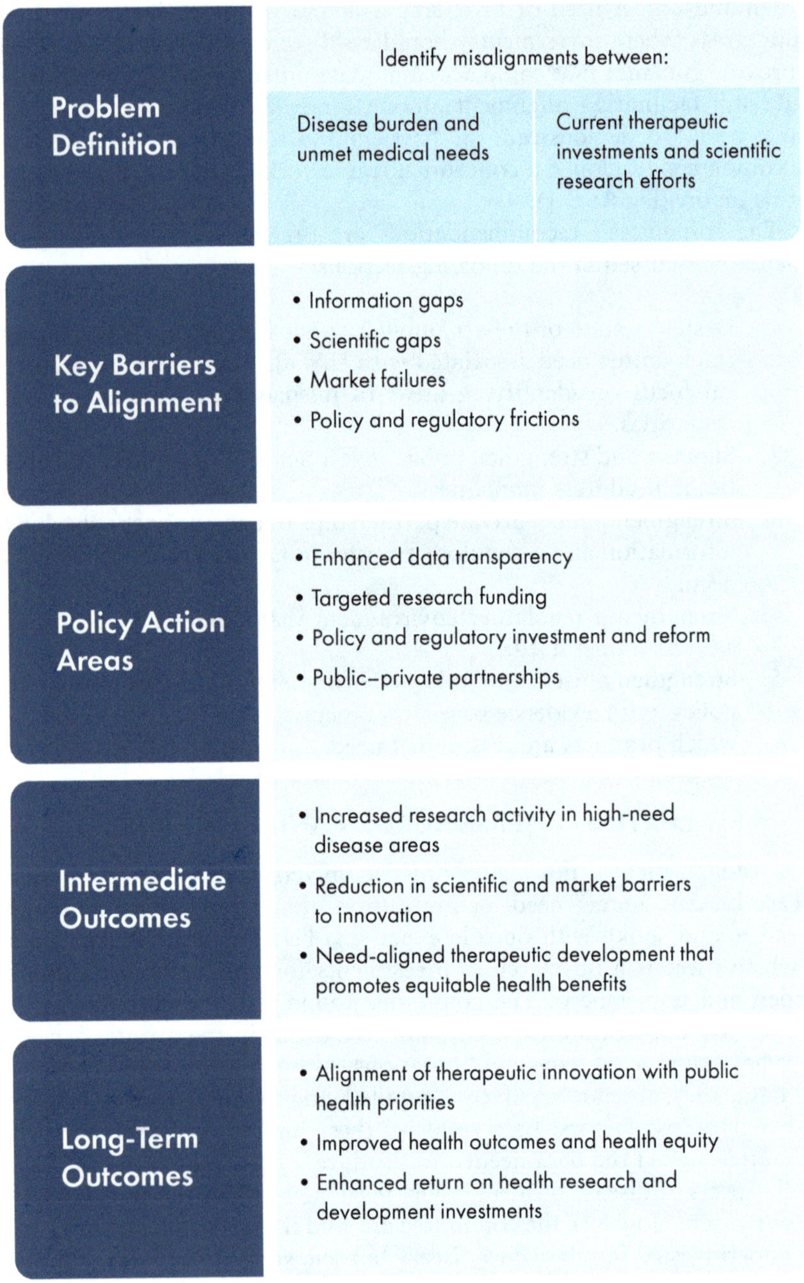

Problem Definition

Identify misalignments between:

Disease burden and unmet medical needs	Current therapeutic investments and scientific research efforts

Key Barriers to Alignment

- Information gaps
- Scientific gaps
- Market failures
- Policy and regulatory frictions

Policy Action Areas

- Enhanced data transparency
- Targeted research funding
- Policy and regulatory investment and reform
- Public–private partnerships

Intermediate Outcomes

- Increased research activity in high-need disease areas
- Reduction in scientific and market barriers to innovation
- Need-aligned therapeutic development that promotes equitable health benefits

Long-Term Outcomes

- Alignment of therapeutic innovation with public health priorities
- Improved health outcomes and health equity
- Enhanced return on health research and development investments

FIGURE S-1 Conceptual framework work aligning investment with therapeutic need.

conditions as headaches, neck and back pain, psoriasis, and gallbladder diseases.[2] The literature sources on private-sector investment, though limited, indicate substantial investment in oncology and neurological disease and suggest underinvestment in cardiovascular disease, immune-related disorders, and maternal and neonatal conditions.

Given the reality that resources are limited and cannot be simultaneously directed toward all health and research needs, a systematic approach is needed to set research priorities and funding allocations to address public health needs. Currently, leaders have imperfect data upon which to make scientifically informed policy judgments. Limitations in the availability of data necessary to assess how investments in therapeutic development align with disease burden and unmet medical need is one factor that contributes to misalignment between investments in therapeutic development and unmet medical need during research prioritization. As a result, public research funds are being allocated each year with insufficient information about the extent to which the investment addresses public health needs.

Conclusion 3-1:[3] *More comprehensive, specific, timely, and accurate data on disease burden, unmet need, and innovation, as well as improved data aggregation, are essential for private and public funders to systematically use measures of disease burden and unmet need when making decisions about funding priorities.*

A publicly accessible, centralized system to aggregate relevant data and track unmet medical needs associated with disease burden would enable more strategic investment of resources and would help policy makers and public and private funding groups better align innovation and investment with public health needs. This system could be used to identify disease areas in which to prioritize investment and to highlight areas of mismatch between investment and disease burden—including both underinvestment in some conditions and overinvestment relative to burden in others. Having access to data on burden, need, and current measures of public and private investment would enable public and private funders to make informed decisions based on their priorities and values. For example, some may prioritize rare, low-prevalence diseases with high individual burden, while others may prioritize diseases with high population burden or high health disparities.

---

[2] See analysis in Chapter 3, "Degree and Patterns of Mismatch Between U.S. Disease Burden and Public and Private Investment in Innovative Therapeutic Development." Terms for diseases and conditions are drawn from the Institute for Health Metrics and Evaluation Global Burden of Disease dataset.

[3] The conclusions in this summary are numbered based on how they present in the chapters of the report.

Developing such a system is challenging. For instance, both burden and unmet need can be interpreted in multiple ways and must be carefully defined in designing this system. Current investments are similarly difficult to assess, especially in the private sector. In addition, while some data are readily available and could be aggregated for this purpose, the committee recognizes that not all the data described in Recommendation 1 are currently or easily accessible. Nevertheless, collecting these data is essential to advancing public health and reducing health disparities. Finally, it is critical that the information collected on evaluating disease burden, unmet need, and the areas of investment be made public for all to use.

Conclusion 3-2: Collecting and aggregating these data requires ongoing stewardship to most effectively address unmet clinical need and reduce health disparities.

Conclusion 3-3: The U.S. government has a responsibility to ensure that timely data on public investment and population health data be made publicly available to support research and strategic investment in areas of unmet need.

Following these conclusions, the committee specifically recommends the following:

Recommendation 1: Congress should establish and fund an interagency consortium charged with tracking and assessing unmet therapeutic need associated with U.S. disease burden and current investments in innovation, with a critical focus on identifying areas of mismatch and reducing health disparities. The consortium should be led by a relevant unit of the Department of Health and Human Services (HHS) as determined by the secretary of HHS.
  This consortium should be charged with the following:
  a. Generate a publicly accessible data repository on disease burden, therapeutic investment, and unmet needs that is updated on a triennial basis and used to generate derivative reports.
  b. Produce a triennial report to Congress on the status of U.S. disease burden, extent of unmet need, and areas in which additional data are needed to reliably assess burden and unmet need. This report should collate, at minimum, for each disease area the current and projected incidence, prevalence, mortality, and disability-adjusted life-years.
  c. Produce a companion assessment of the most reliable current estimates of investments from the public and private sectors for each therapeutic area, including public-sector funding by type

and amount; private-sector investments; stage of the development pipeline for emerging treatments (e.g., drug discovery, preclinical research, clinical trials, regulatory review and approval, post-approval surveillance); the number, phase, and status of clinical trials; and sources of funding.

d. Identify areas in which additional research is needed to provide any missing information for each item above and recommend ways, such as statutory requirements or surveys, by which the data could be gathered for subsequent reports.

To implement this recommendation most effectively, this consortium should involve cross-agency and disciplinary collaborators, including the Food and Drug Administration (FDA), NIH, Advanced Research Projects Agency for Health (ARPA-H), Centers for Disease Control and Prevention (CDC), the Office of the Assistant Secretary for Planning and Evaluation, as well as many other federal agencies and key partners, such as the Patient-Centered Outcomes Research Institute and industry organizations. It is important for this consortium not only to collate these data but also analyze and synthesize the data, including identifying gaps and ways to fill them. For example, given the challenge of collecting information on private industry investments, companies may need incentives to share or disclose some of these data that are not now publicly available. One way of collecting this information could be through a survey of pharmaceutical and biotech companies, which, while imperfect, could gather a useful sampling of data to gain insight into private investment in therapeutic development. The collecting of these data could be incentivized by allowing early access to updated datasets and reports to private and public companies that have contributed to the repository, which would provide a valuable, precompetitive output that companies could use to inform business decisions.

REASONS THERE IS A MISMATCH BETWEEN INVESTMENT, DISEASE BURDEN, AND UNMET NEED AND RECOMMENDATIONS TO ADDRESS THEM

Accelerating medical breakthroughs and enabling individualized screening, prevention, treatment, and care for all depends on the entire innovation pipeline from basic science through clinical trials, regulatory approvals, and postmarketing evidence generation and implementation. A barrier in any one of these areas can slow or halt innovation. Although there are many challenges and barriers in drug development broadly, the committee focused on the reasons for underlying mismatches between research and development (R&D) investments and areas of unmet need. The committee identified two high-level factors that underlie the observed mismatch: scientific challenges and market forces.

Scientific Challenges

A lack of understanding of underlying pathophysiology is a fundamental barrier to therapeutic development for many diseases, such as Alzheimer's disease and mental health conditions. Life science investors and industry scientists depend on advances in basic and preclinical biomedical research, areas that have traditionally been funded largely by NIH, to direct their attention and funding. The committee also identified scientific challenges in measuring outcomes for some conditions, such as chronic pain, when measures are subjective, highly variable, or difficult to characterize. Similarly, a lack of plausible surrogate endpoints in some disease areas prevents drug developers from using the accelerated approval pathway, which is designed to bring therapeutics to market faster on the condition that they complete postmarketing studies to confirm clinical benefits. The committee found that investment in preclinical biomedical research is essential to driving innovation in disease areas with significant burden and unmet needs.

These investments in research must be informed by the comprehensive system to track and assess disease burden and unmet needs, as outlined in Recommendation 1. Congress plays a key role in defining the parameters of public investment in medical research by setting appropriations among the NIH's institutes and centers. Information about burden and unmet need should be incorporated at key points of decision making and should serve as a key input for determining congressional appropriations and funding decisions at NIH and other federal agencies.

However, considering the burden and unmet need should not be limited to appropriations. Such considerations should be explicitly integrated throughout the research funding process, from program development to grant review criteria, ensuring that unmet need is considered alongside scientific merit in grant mechanisms. This holistic approach would help align incentives by encouraging investigators to consider unmet needs early in the research process. When funding agencies elevate the goal of addressing unmet need as a priority, researchers are more likely to develop studies to target these areas, leading to better alignment of public and private investment in medical research with public health needs.

Recommendation 2: Funders of biomedical research should consider disease burden and unmet need when setting research priorities and directing funding. Specific actions to ensure both population health needs and scientific merit are considered in grant funding mechanisms include:

a. Congress should consider disease burden and unmet needs when setting appropriations to agencies that fund biomedical research, including in allocating funding among National Institutes of Health institutes and centers.

b. Public and private funders should develop targeted research funding opportunities specific to diseases with the highest mismatch of burden and unmet need, including funding opportunities for innovative methods to enable the development of therapeutic products and new biomarkers for diagnostic test development in these areas.

c. Public and private funders should allocate funds for the development and validation of new biomarkers and surrogate endpoints for diseases with high unmet medical need.

d. Public and private funders should provide funding for studies of disease epidemiology or basic science for areas where there is a critical need for understanding the mechanisms of disease.

e. Public and private funders should include explicit criteria that include, but are not limited to, unmet need and disease burden for evaluating proposals in the grant review process and funding decisions.

In addition to directing investments in biomedical science toward unmet needs, it is important to ensure a robust infrastructure exists for regulatory review to facilitate drug approval and surveillance in these areas. Although FDA sometimes is cited as a barrier to innovation, the committee did not find evidence to support the claim that misalignment between investment and unmet need was attributable to action or inaction from FDA. In fact, FDA has several ongoing programs to drive innovation in much-needed areas. These programs generally fall into three categories: (1) efforts to encourage investment to address unmet need; (2) efforts to address broad scientific challenges, improve coordination, and encourage data generation to address unmet need; and (3) efforts to facilitate and expedite development and review to address unmet need. After extensively reviewing the evidence around these programs, the committee made the following conclusion:

Conclusion 5-3: Additional resources are needed for FDA programs that successfully support endpoint development and validation, innovative trial design, and the resolution of other broad scientific challenges that impede drug development for unmet needs, as well as programs designed to support communication between sponsors and FDA to quickly resolve challenges arising in specific development programs.

Recommendation 6: To maintain the appropriateness of Food and Drug Administration (FDA) programs that expedite the development and review of therapies in areas of unmet need, including the accelerated approval program, FDA should generously use its authority to impose postmarket study requirements, ensure that required postmarket studies are appropriately designed to confirm clinical benefit, and strictly enforce postmarket study requirements. The following steps will support these goals:

a. FDA should ensure that confirmatory studies are well designed to evaluate clinical benefit, and should prespecify the study results that will be deemed acceptable for conversion to traditional approval.

b. FDA should continue recent efforts to ensure that confirmatory studies are underway before approval is granted, making exceptions only in extreme cases.

c. If concerns about timely study completion arise during progress reports, then FDA and the sponsor should determine the steps needed to address barriers; any modification to study requirements should prioritize ensuring rigor.

d. For drugs whose studies fail to confirm clinical benefits following flexible approval, FDA should use its authority to rapidly withdraw approval.

e. FDA should lead an effort, in collaboration with the National Institutes of Health and the Centers for Medicare & Medicaid Services, to enable more efficient conversion of unvalidated endpoints to validated endpoints to advance therapeutic innovation.

FDA currently exercises a great deal of regulatory flexibility, including beyond that offered in existing programs, such as through the use of accelerated approval. Regulatory flexibility can be appropriate as long as there is an expectation that clinical benefit will be confirmed within a reasonable time frame after approval and that those expectations are enforced by requiring rigorous confirmatory studies to be completed in a timely manner and rapidly acting on their results.

While greater regulatory flexibility can speed access to *promising* therapeutics, what patients truly need are *safe* and *effective* therapeutics. Thus, flexibility must be balanced against the importance of maintaining strong regulatory standards. For example, regulatory flexibility may be unavoidable for certain rare diseases, where it is nearly impossible to meet standard expectations. However, regulatory flexibility that allows for approval when trials fail to show clinical benefit raise a number of concerns, including the possibility of misleading patients, inhibiting the development of the information necessary to guide clinical decision making, and impeding the conduct of clinical trials for other drugs that may be more efficacious, both by discouraging further trial participation and influencing expectations around standard-of-care comparators.

Occasionally, FDA has extended its flexibility by wide margins to approve drugs despite substantial uncertainty about their benefit, including drugs that failed to meet prespecified endpoints in pivotal or confirmatory studies. Despite this expansive current flexibility, FDA faces frequent pressure to go even further. Because weak approval standards harm all patients, and FDA is a public health agency that must consider what is in the best interests of populations, the committee does not recommend approaches that would extend the agency's flexibility in drug approvals beyond what is currently permitted.

> Recommendation 7: To ensure that regulatory flexibility is exercised in a manner that promotes the approval of drugs that are both safe and effective, the Food and Drug Administration (FDA) should uphold strong regulatory approval standards. When FDA exercises flexibility, whether through accelerated approval or outside that pathway, the agency should require rigorous, timely confirmatory studies.

For FDA to maintain many of the existing pathways and initiatives that address areas of therapeutic need, the agency requires appropriate funding and staffing, and agency personnel need appropriate job security. FDA is a staff-intensive agency, with approximately 80 percent of its budget devoted to personnel costs needed to appropriately recruit and retain individuals with the expertise needed to regulate the nation's food, drugs, and medical devices. Expanding the FDA workforce would allow the agency to keep pace with technological and scientific breakthroughs. However, FDA has faced a number of concerning staff disruptions recently—including layoffs, retirements, and departures—threatening the agency's ability to manage its intensive workload and advance innovative approaches.

> *Conclusion 5-8: Support for innovation in the pre- and postmarket settings requires a well-resourced regulatory environment, including attracting and retaining FDA staff with the necessary experience and expertise for innovative technologies.*

> Recommendation 8: Congress should authorize a significant expansion of Food and Drug Administration (FDA) staffing and consistent resources to support the implementation of Recommendations 6 and 7, and especially to ensure that FDA has sufficient resources to monitor and enforce requirements for postmarketing surveillance and drug evaluation research.

Market Forces

Many factors contribute to investment decisions, but given the involvement of for-profit firms in the financing of drug development, expectations about returns on investment are of major importance. For some disease areas, market forces discourage drug developers from investing in or pursuing therapeutics because the potential earnings or return on investment from a new therapy are too low to justify a further investment in R&D. Rare diseases, by definition, are those that affect small populations; in the United States the cutoff point is typically 200,000 people. The market for these therapies is small, and so for many years the return on investment has been generally considered to be too small for market development. Most rare diseases fall into the categories of ultrarare and hyperrare diseases, making the market for these drugs extremely small.

A second factor that affects calculations for therapeutic investment is the duration of treatment. For drug developers, chronic disease states—where the duration of therapy is unlimited—offer greater opportunities to profit than do acute conditions, on average. This can create a financial disincentive for investors considering returns for curative therapies that have short treatment times.

One potential strategy to address market forces and promote therapeutic development is to use public–private partnerships (PPPs), which can be particularly beneficial for innovation in areas where cost and risk sharing are valuable, such as novel drug target discovery, biomarker testing, or preclinical development models. The committee identified three key areas of unmet needs where PPPs could address innovation challenges:

1. Expand the development of better diagnostics, which is an area that is sometimes difficult for investment from the private sector because of market failures and payment structures for diagnostic tests.
2. Limit situations where therapies that are effective and that meet an unmet need are taken off the market or where assets demonstrating early signs of efficacy are shelved before making it to market.
3. Provide an avenue for the development of drugs for diseases where there exists no economic incentive for the private sector to develop therapeutics.

Conclusion 5-9: Strengthening and expanding public–private partnerships, such as the Network for Excellence in Neuroscience Clinical Trials, the National Cancer Institute Experimental Therapeutics program, and Bridging Interventional Development Gaps, could help address innovation challenges for therapeutic areas with unmet needs.

In addition to recommending additional support for existing PPP models that have shown promise in addressing gaps in the drug development pipelines, the committee makes the following recommendation:

> Recommendation 3: U.S. federal scientific agencies with congressionally authorized nonprofit organizations, such as the Foundation for the National Institutes of Health, Centers for Disease Control and Prevention Foundation, Reagan-Udall Foundation, and Henry M. Jackson Foundation for the Advancement of Military Medicine, should increase use of their nonprofits in order to focus on building public–private partnerships in areas of mismatch between unmet need (encompassing both therapeutics and diagnostics) and innovation.

Despite the successes of existing PPPs and the potential to expand these to enhance innovation in needed therapeutic areas, several barriers exist within the United States to developing more PPPs. First, PPPs are often initiated by federal agencies seeking to expand therapeutic development in a specific area. Such agencies approach private firms about entering a PPP to contribute financial support or in-kind resources and assets. In the areas of high unmet need with low economic incentives for the private sector, these PPPs are often focused on shelved assets that companies have developed but chosen not to pursue. However, the federal agencies do not always have insight into what shelved assets exist and therefore are unable to approach companies about developing these assets. Therefore, having an independent organization house a searchable repository of assets to which companies voluntarily submit information could help overcome this barrier. To safeguard proprietary information, such a repository might not be publicly available, but it could be viewed by federal agencies and other foundations and nonprofits that apply for access. Although it likely would not provide a complete list of shelved assets, it would be a start for advancing PPPs in areas of unmet need and where the market does not support further innovation with a specific compound.

> Recommendation 4: The National Institutes of Health should work with a neutral third-party entity to set up a searchable repository of assets no longer under development by commercial sponsors to be shared with foundations and other entities to take forward for testing. The information in the repository could be voluntarily provided by companies potentially looking to enter public–private partnerships to develop an asset.

Finally, there is an urgent need to better align payer coverage and reimbursement policies to ensure market access for products addressing unmet need. Specifically, aligning reimbursement policy with evidence-based therapeutic value could create stronger incentives for investment in products targeting unmet need and also provide patients with improved access to these products. Research indicates that pharmaceutical companies respond to financial incentives and direct innovation efforts toward areas with the greatest financial incentives, so by aligning reimbursement policy with therapeutic value (i.e., how much clinical benefit a drug offers), investment would shift toward developing products with demonstrated clinical benefit addressing unmet needs.

Reimbursement policy through public (e.g., Medicare and Medicaid) and private plans (employer sponsored and individual market health plans) determines both whether a novel drug is covered and, if covered, the amount paid by beneficiaries. Disincentives for innovation can occur if novel drugs that address unmet needs are not covered or are covered but not readily accessible by patients because of access restrictions or cost-sharing that is unaffordable for patients. In addition, providing high coverage and payment for therapies without demonstrated clinical benefit or substantive innovation reduces the potential of reimbursement policy to incentivize the development of high-value treatments. Aligning reimbursement policy with evidence-based value and unmet need is key to this committee's aims of promoting innovation and addressing unmet need.

A revised approach to reimbursement policy could help address innovation incentives for therapeutical development by linking pricing to evidence-based value assessments that incorporate clinical effectiveness and patient perspectives. Many other countries, including the UK and Germany, offer useful models for this approach of prioritizing payment for new therapies that address unmet need and limiting reimbursement for products that offer marginal improvements or whose clinical benefit remains unproven, although the details of these programs would need to be adapted for the United States. Linking pricing to value is also important because prioritizing payment for high-value innovative therapies (while limiting overpaying for lower value treatments) could make more resources available for improving coverage for effective therapies.

Conclusion 5-10: If public and private payer reimbursement policies were more aligned with evidence of product value and the extent to which a drug addresses unmet medical need, greater innovation would occur in therapeutic areas with high unmet need.

Conclusion 5-11: Congressional action is needed to more directly tie prices and public insurance reimbursement for novel drugs that address unmet need to evidence-supported measures of value or impact.

Recommendation 9: Congress should reform the statutory framework that regulates public reimbursement for novel drugs to better align reimbursement rates with evidence of clinical benefit as compared with existing therapeutic alternatives, if any. This could include:

a. Expand the Centers for Medicare & Medicaid Services' authority and capacity to negotiate prices beyond the scope of the Inflation Reduction Act to account for the value of the drug relative to alternatives or a standard of care, including the extent to which it addresses unmet need.

b. For drugs with negotiated prices, set reimbursement terms that maximize patient access through more favorable cost-sharing, robust formulary coverage, and more tailored application of utilization management tools (e.g., prior authorization, step-therapy, and quantity limits).

In addition to the broader market challenges for therapeutics, there are specific challenges that must be addressed for one-time, curative, or regenerative medicine therapies. Novel one-time or limited duration curative therapies have been developed in recent years, but it has often proved difficult for them to reach patients. Recent examples have included treatments for hepatitis C, lymphomas and leukemias, beta thalassemia, and sickle cell anemia. With new developments in cell and gene therapies in recent years, the number of such therapies is increasing. It is important that these therapies continue to be developed—some are highly effective and innovative, but the market and access barriers are significant.

The benefit designs and utilization management employed by many insurance payers in the United States make it difficult for clinicians, individual patients, manufacturers, and innovators to navigate coverage and patient access for very high-priced drugs. This has resulted in lower or no access to certain drugs, depending on insurance coverage and even geography (e.g., variation by states among Medicaid insured populations).

Recent evidence also suggests that as commercial products have underperformed, new investments in cell and gene therapies and curative therapies are being challenged, and drug developers have begun to retreat from this market, despite the exceptional benefits of these products for patients (especially those with very rare diseases). To improve affordability and access for patients and to sustain investments in these needed innovative treatments, novel solutions for payment, coverage, and market access for drug developers, payers, and patients are needed.

Conclusion 4-1: Innovative therapies are emerging for rare diseases and other complex conditions, offering a potential for cure. However, the fragmented payment system within the United States is a barrier to patient access, resulting in underinvestment in developing curative therapies. The current U.S. market and policy environment is unprepared to manage these one-time, very high-cost therapies. There is a need for a clearer reimbursement structure for innovators developing these high-cost curative treatments.

Recommendation 11: Congress should support the development of a negotiation and access model for one-time curative therapies to ensure access for patients and market access for innovators of novel therapies.

To begin this work, Congress could instruct an organization or agency, such as the Medicare Payment Advisory Commission or the Medicaid and CHIP Payment and Access Commission, to study and develop recommendations for legislation to create a new program addressing the unique deficiencies of the nation's current insurance system in enabling access to curative therapies.

CONCLUSION

Therapeutic innovation in the United States has powered medical innovation around the world, but unmet needs remain. Current research prioritization is done without the data on disease burden, unmet need, and investment needed to guide decision making. A robust, timely, accessible data system is key to implementing recommended changes in policies and practice that can deliver better health outcomes from the resources invested in innovation. With better information on disease burden and unmet need, we can make more strategic investments in basic science. These strategic investments will drive scientific discoveries that enable more efficient clinical research that—when accompanied by aligned market incentives—can bring to market effective therapies that address critical unmet needs.

1

Introduction

The development of novel therapeutics involves complex decisions about where to focus resources and investment. In principle, investment in therapeutic development should target the diseases and conditions with the highest unmet need and burden on societies and individuals. However, both public and private funders and investors developing therapeutics consider disease burden and unmet need in the context of myriad competing considerations and goals, such as limited funding; balancing advances in basic, translational, and clinical science; advocacy from patient groups; the likelihood of regulatory approval; payer reimbursement; market competition; and overall return-on-investment. These competing practical and financial priorities do not always align with unmet needs, underscoring the critical question of to what extent investments in new treatments correspond to the areas of greatest unmet need.

Furthermore, how to fairly allocate resources for drug development among potential beneficiaries involves ethical considerations and value judgments, about which there is not universal agreement and for which a multitude of defensible approaches exist. Because resources are limited and must be balanced with development in other sectors of society, and because public and private actors have different priorities, risk tolerance, and responsibilities, fairly allocating resources for drug development is a critical issue with multiple potential approaches (Millum, 2024).

Investments in therapeutic development have substantially increased the number of drugs entering the market, particularly in the last 2 decades (Austin and Hayford, 2021). This period has seen breakthroughs that have improved, even transformed, patient care—including targeted cancer therapies like Gleevec and Herceptin, the development of novel cell and gene therapies, and highly effective GLP-1 receptor agonists. These advances represent significant innovation, but not all drugs fit that category. Studies conducted in the United States, Canada, and Europe indicate that many drugs that received marketing approval over the past 50 years were not considered pharmacologically or therapeutically innovative or did not demonstrate substantive improvements in efficacy or safety over the standard of care. The incentive for incremental improvements is not always aligned with their actual benefit for society. Some drugs are reimbursed at high prices despite demonstrating only marginal improvements (Austin and Hayford, 2021; Darrow et al., 2020; Kaitin et al., 1991; Kergall et al., 2021; Morgan et al., 2005; Rodwin et al., 2021; Wieseler et al., 2019). Although, even modest improvements in delivery, route of administration, or frequency of administration are important as they can enhance adherence, improve health outcomes, and address unmet need. In addition, the development of "me-too" or follow-on drugs, though not innovative, can increase competition and lower prices, or expand indications to new patient populations. However, there is a role for both innovation and incremental improvements in therapeutic developments that address unmet need. Investments in research and development (R&D) for innovation as well as incremental improvements could be better aligned with disease burden and unmet need in the United States (see Chapter 4).

In addition, many diseases and conditions continue to cause high disease burden and have substantial unmet need. Some diseases and conditions have no available therapies, and oftentimes existing, approved therapies are only modestly effective or have important safety risks. Unmet needs are often exacerbated by health disparities across population groups. These disparities are commonly associated with differences between groups in disease occurrence, health insurance coverage, care affordability, and access and quality of health care services and treatments. The current system of drug development needs adjusting to better align our investments in therapeutics with areas of unmet need.

PHARMACEUTICAL DEVELOPMENT AND THE DRUG DEVELOPMENT CYCLE

The development cycle for drugs is a lengthy process. Drug development typically begins with basic science research. Although basic science research is conducted by private companies, much is done by investigators at academic centers with funding from the National Institutes of Health (NIH) or other public sources. Translational research begins to build on basic science research and identify human applications. Once the research is advanced enough to identify potential product applications, which can be a difficult hurdle to clear in order to attract private investment, universities license promising technology to private companies to support technology transfer, or scientists may form biotech start-ups, requiring some early investment of capital. Occasionally, academic scientists will create public–private partnerships (PPPs) to advance their products, especially for products that may be perceived as not having a profitable market. Preclinical development focuses on *in vitro* and *in vivo* studies, manufacturing process development, and toxicology studies. Once initial studies are completed for a promising drug candidate, preclinical data are compiled for an investigational new drug (IND) application to seek permission from the Food and Drug Administration (FDA) to begin testing an experimental drug in humans. An IND filing is a key milestone for drug development and for investors. The drug then undergoes a series of clinical trials to determine safety and efficacy, while in parallel the manufacturing process is refined and improved for commercialization.

Phase I through phase III clinical trials involve progressively larger patient populations and become increasingly expensive and time consuming, requiring substantial capital investment primarily from venture capital firms or established pharmaceutical companies. Clinical trial data are submitted in a new drug application or a biologics license application to FDA for approval, which is another key milestone in drug development. In the commercial and postmarketing phases, pricing and reimbursement negotiations occur with payers, and product revenue begins to deliver return on investment. Sometimes there are phase IV studies or studies to collect clinical trial data for postapproval confirmation of short- and long-term benefits and safety, or expansions for other indications. (See NASEM, 2022, 2023, for further descriptions of this drug development cycle.)

Drug development requires a substantial investment of time (often over a decade from initial discovery to market approval) and money (approximately $1.1 billion per new molecular entity, including the costs of successful R&D programs as well as failures) (Sertkaya et al., 2024; Wouters and Kesselheim, 2024). Most candidate drugs fail in clinical trials; it has been estimated that approximately 1 in 10 assets entering phase I trials ultimately meets the statutory standard of safety and effectiveness to support approval (Austin and Hayford, 2021). However, the cost of R&D and the probability of product success varies by disease category (Sertkaya et al., 2024). Given the high level of investment required and the high risk of the pharmaceutical development process, decision making about where to invest time and capital is critical and occurs with each phase of the process from discovery through approval. Many factors contribute to financial and personnel investment decisions, but whether capital for R&D comes from venture capital firms or established pharmaceutical companies, the entities are profit seeking, so expectations about the timing and amount of returns on investment are of utmost importance.

To aid in decision making, companies use various types of analysis. For example, net present value forecasts are used to analyze the potential return on investment, accounting for the likely volume of use, the net pricing of and expected reimbursement for the envisioned product, and the duration of its patents or market exclusivity. Drivers for investment decisions also include such factors as the size of the target patient population, disease severity, profile of existing competing products, and more. Unmet need and disease burden can factor into these assessments when accounting for market trends, gaps, and competitive products, but a lot of decision making is related to return on investment, which can leave gaps where resources are not directed toward some areas of unmet need.

The United States prizes the role it plays in technological innovation and has been a powerhouse of innovation in pharmaceutical development. However, the level of investment does not always yield the desired health outcomes and high-value therapeutics. To better address U.S. health needs, it is important to direct investments that can create larger health care gains without sacrificing financial returns. Recognizing the value of innovation, the committee's goal is to better align investment with disease burden and unmet need.

COMMITTEE TASK AND APPROACH

Several years ago, a group was convened to discuss health care costs and proposed strategies to reduce costs without harming patients. During those conversations, questions were raised about whether investments in therapeutics are made where they are most needed. However, given the relative lack of data for quantifying public and private investments in therapeutic innovation, it became clear that there was an opportunity to delve more deeply into that question. Therefore, with support from Gates Ventures and the Peterson Center on Healthcare, the National Academies of Sciences, Engineering, and Medicine (the National Academies) formed the Committee on Strategies to Better Align Investments in Innovations for Therapeutic Development with Disease Burden and Unmet Needs. The sponsors charged the committee to develop strategies to improve investment in innovation to reduce gaps in disease burden and unmet need (Box 1-1).

The Committee's Interpretation of the Charge

The committee approached its statement of task with the overall goal to design policies that would lead society to invest in innovation (including public and private investments) up to the point where the marginal cost equals the expected marginal social benefit of those investments. In other words, U.S. policies should help ensure that all cost-effective innovations

BOX 1-1
Statement of Task

An ad hoc committee of the National Academies of Sciences, Engineering, and Medicine will examine the current degree and patterns of alignment or mismatch between innovation in developing novel therapies and unmet needs associated with U.S. disease burden (including high-impact, low-frequency diseases as well as highly prevalent conditions). The committee will recommend strategies to spur and facilitate increased innovation to address unmet needs and reduce health disparities. In addition to reviewing the published literature and publicly available information sources, the committee will identify and engage appropriate stakeholders, including relevant federal agencies (e.g., NIH, Advanced Research Projects Agency for Health, FDA, Centers for Medicare & Medicaid Services), the academic/professional community of researchers and clinicians, private industry, and patient/consumer groups, to gain their perspectives as input to committee deliberations. Based on the information gathered, the committee will identify the challenges, opportunities, and responsibilities in building both public and private capacity for innovation in therapeutic development and ensuring broad, equitable access to safe and effective novel therapies.

The committee will address three overarching questions:

1. How well or poorly is the current pipeline of public and private innovations and investments in developing new therapies aligned with the actual burden of illness, injury, and disability in the United States?
2. What changes in policy, finance, regulation, and other influences would help achieve better alignment to address unmet needs and reduce health disparities?
3. Are there unmet needs that should be prioritized within the proposed changes?

Specifically, the committee will:

1. Describe the current U.S. disease burden, with consideration of such topics as:
   a. The total burden of illness, injury, and disability in the United States by therapeutic area, including high-impact, low-frequency diseases as well as highly prevalent conditions
   b. Disease areas with the greatest unmet need for effective therapies (excluding unmet need caused by lack of access to existing therapies)

continued

BOX 1-1 Continued

   c. The effect of comorbidities and downstream outcomes for unmet needs on health care spending (e.g., mental health conditions)

   d. Variations in burden across different populations (e.g., age, race, gender, socioeconomic status, payer mix)

2. Characterize the degree and patterns of mismatch between U.S. disease burden and public and private innovation in therapeutic development, with consideration of topics such as:

   a. The portion of the disease burden for which the standard of care is inadequate and for which outcomes could potentially be improved by innovative therapies

   b. Potential proxies for determining innovation efforts by disease area (e.g., clinical trials, total funding, novelty and effectiveness of new therapies)

   c. The areas of mismatch for which remedies could have the greatest effect on U.S. disease burden and health equity

3. Describe the challenges in better aligning innovations in therapeutic development with disease burden and unmet needs, with consideration of topics such as:

   a. Decision making by for-profit and private-sector developers for investments in innovation, including perceptions of potential risks and returns (e.g., drivers of variation that inform measures of investments across therapeutic areas and needs, such as net present value)

   b. The greatest challenges to overcome in the different stages of development for neglected disease areas (e.g., basic and translational science, clinical trials)

   c. The role of public investment in biomedical research, and how that investment is used in the development of novel therapies

4. Propose strategies informed by population needs, society costs, and assessments of potential risks and returns to better align both public and private investments in innovations in therapeutic development with disease burden and unmet needs. The committee may make recommendations to a variety of actors, such as federal agencies and Congress, the pharmaceutical industry, and private philanthropy, with consideration of topics such as:

   a. Ways to better use existing policies and programs to incentivize high-value innovation

   b. Potential new policies to facilitate greater investment in innovation to address unmet need as well as to discourage practices that impede innovation or competition

---

BOX 1-1 Continued

c. The potential role of public–private partnerships and pre-competitive collaboration
d. Potential innovations in regulatory science and practices
e. Lessons learned from rapid innovations during the COVID-19 pandemic
f. Potential new policies to ensure equitable patient access to innovative therapies that effectively address unmet needs

---

can make it to market, and that resources are not being spent on projects that are expected to have little benefit in terms of saving lives and improving health. The marginal cost part of this equation is relatively straightforward, although it is challenging to get such data in practice, as one can theoretically approach cost as the sum of private and public investment. However, the expected social benefit of these investments is much more complicated. This social benefit depends on the estimated reduction in disease burden that the R&D investment could cause and on a judgment about how to value that disease burden reduction, which includes challenging ethical questions about how to value different kinds of health gains and inequality reductions. While there have been efforts to quantify social benefit as a monetary value, such valuations are beyond the scope of this report.

As discussed in detail in Chapter 2, there are various ways to measure disease burden and unmet need, depending on values and priorities. (See Box 1-2 for definitions for key terms used throughout this report.) Therefore, the committee does not prescribe a single approach for calculating disease burden and unmet need nor does it provide a definitive list of diseases or therapeutic areas where investments should be directed. Instead, the committee sought to provide a framework for accomplishing such a task. The committee reviewed current evidence relating to mismatch between U.S. disease burden and investments, as described in Chapter 3; however, much of this report is dedicated to advancing a clearer understanding of the contours of assessing burden and unmet need and developing guidance for conducting this assessment systematically and on an ongoing basis. In addition, disease exemplars are used throughout the report to highlight areas of mismatch between U.S. disease burden and public and private innovation in therapeutic development. These exemplars are not meant to be an exhaustive list of areas of mismatch but instead highlight some of the challenges in our current system to align investments in therapeutic development with U.S. disease burden and unmet need.

BOX 1-2
Key Terminology Used in This Report

The definitions of some of the key terms in the statement of task, such as disease burden and unmet need, are the subject of debate among researchers and are also shifting. Acknowledging the differences in terms used by different researchers and stakeholder groups, the committee opted to use the terms as defined below. Please see the referenced section for a more in-depth analysis of the terminology used throughout the report.

Disease burden: "The term *burden of disease* generally describes the total, cumulative consequences of a defined disease" (Hessel, 2008, p. 94) and in some cases is broadly inclusive of health, social aspects, and costs to society. Disease burden encompasses the health consequences of disease occurrence, including morbidity and mortality, and can also include the effects on the quality of life of individuals and costs to society (see Chapter 2).

Unmet need: A medical condition or disease for which there are either: (1) no existing clinically effective therapeutic treatment options, (2) existing therapeutic solutions with limited effectiveness, or (3) existing effective therapies that have limited effect owing to access or adherence challenges.

Innovation: Novel therapeutics that are cost-effective and result in substantial improvements in health outcomes, higher quality of life, and higher benefit-to-risk ratio, as compared to the existing standard of care.

Chronic disease: A condition that "last[s] 1 year or more and require[s] ongoing medical attention, limit[s] activities of daily living, or both" (CDC, 2024a).

Health equity: "The state in which everyone has a fair and just opportunity to attain their highest level of health" (CDC, 2025). Achieving this requires focused and ongoing societal efforts to address historical and contemporary injustices; overcome economic, social, and other obstacles to health and health care; and eliminate preventable health disparities (CDC, 2025).

Health inequities: Particular "types of health disparities that stem from unfair and unjust systems, policies, and practices and limit access to the opportunities and resources needed to live the healthiest life possible" (CDC, 2024b).

Social determinants of health: "The nonmedical factors that influence health outcomes…[and] the conditions in which people are born, grow, work, live, and age, and the wider set of forces and systems shaping the conditions of daily life" (CDC, 2024b). These forces (e.g., racism, climate, socioeconomic status, education) and systems include "economic policies, development agendas, social norms, social policies, and political systems," along with workplace conditions (CDC, 2024b).

The committee focuses its analysis on U.S. disease burden and U.S. investment in accordance with the statement of task. However, the committee acknowledges that therapeutic research and development is a global endeavor. As such, global disease burden likely contributes to investment decisions in the U.S. market, particularly among multinational companies or organizations focused on global health. Moreover, research occurring in other countries can contribute to therapeutic innovations for American patients without being reflected in U.S. investments. While quantifying these factors' effects on the mismatch of investment and unmet need in the United States is beyond the scope of this committee, it is important to recognize that the international context is intertwined with U.S. therapeutic funding and innovation.

The committee found that the concept of access is intimately linked with both therapeutic innovation and unmet need. For example, "a back-of-the-envelope calculation suggests that U.S. consumers account for about 64 to 78 percent of total pharmaceutical profits" (Goldman and Lakdawalla, 2018, p. 4), and the drug pricing and market access environment is a major determinant of product success. Therefore, to the extent that drug pricing and access affect innovation, the committee considered this to be within its scope. On the other hand, while the committee recognizes that unmet need is often driven by broader social, economic, and behavioral determinants that influence patient access and the appropriate use of existing therapeutics, an adequate assessment of the policies and practices that address these determinants was beyond the scope of this report, as indicated in the statement of task. However, the effects of these factors on access and health outcomes have been the subject of considerable attention elsewhere in the literature, including recent National Academies reports (NASEM, 2018, 2019, 2023).

The committee thought carefully about whether medical devices, preventatives (e.g., vaccines), and diagnostics were in scope for this report. The committee considered medical devices to be out of scope for its charge given that the regulatory and reimbursement mechanisms differ from those for drugs and including these devices would have expanded the scope too broadly for the committee to address comprehensively within the given time frame. However, the committee recognizes that there are unique considerations for diagnostics that merit further discussion within the scope of this report, such as when therapeutic innovation is particularly limited by a lack of diagnostic innovation. Some conditions would benefit from more granular distinctions in the patient population afforded by better diagnostics, which could allow for more targeted therapies, as well as enhanced efficiency in generating evidence of safety and efficacy. In certain conditions for which early detection and treatment is essential, such as degenerative diseases, novel diagnostics to accurately provide a timely patient diagnosis could result in better therapeutics and fewer unmet needs. Therefore, although pharmaceuticals were the primary focus of the report, diagnostics are mentioned throughout the report where a lack of significant investment in innovation for the development of novel diagnostics serves as a barrier to aligning therapeutic innovation with unmet need and disease burden.

Similarly, this report does not concentrate on vaccines and other preventatives, although preventatives can be critical for addressing disease burden or unmet need. Even though preventatives, medical devices, and such treatments as physical or behavioral therapy were determined to be out of scope for this report, they are often intertwined with therapeutic innovation and it is important to recognize that pharmacological therapies are not the only, or necessarily the best, way to address disease burden or unmet medical need in many cases.

Committee Approach

The Committee on Strategies to Better Align Investments in Innovations for Therapeutic Development with Disease Burden and Unmet Needs consisted of 16 members with a broad range of expertise, including health economics, data science, epidemiology, health policy, biomedical/pharmaceutical sciences, therapeutic development (including those with experience in the biopharmaceutical industry and the investment community), regulatory oversight, health law, bioethics, social and behavioral sciences, clinical care, and health disparities. Appendix B provides brief biographies of the committee members and staff.

The committee deliberated during seven hybrid meetings, many working group calls, and multiple ad hoc meetings between March 2024 and March 2025. Additionally, the committee held three virtual public webinars and invited speakers to offer comments or make presentations to inform the committee's deliberations. Speakers provided valuable input on a broad range of topics, including investment decision making, data and artificial intelligence, regulatory barriers and solutions, and more. Appendix A includes public session agendas, and Appendix D provides more information about the study's methods.

The committee also completed an extensive search of the peer-reviewed literature and the gray literature, including publications by private organizations, advocacy groups, and government entities. In addition, the committee established an online system to collect perspectives from patients and patient groups, clinicians, investors, regulators, policy makers, federal agencies, entrepreneurs, inventors, innovators, and researchers. This "call for perspectives" was posted on the project website, announced at all public meetings, and shared with project sponsors; it included a survey of questions covering patient experiences, clinical insights, investment, regulatory issues, research challenges and solutions, and more.

As noted in this committee's meeting timeline, the majority of the committee's deliberations as well as the writing of this report occurred in a different policy environment from the one into which it is being released. The federal policy landscape for biomedical research is in the midst of a rapidly evolving and unprecedented period of change, altering the federal funding architecture upon which the innovation ecosystem has operated for the past several decades. Despite the uncertainty that accompanies this dramatic period of change, the committee maintains the strong position that alignment of investment in innovation with unmet need is an essential and persistent goal and presents recommendations accordingly. Public investment in research and related regulatory activities is incredibly efficient. For example, for every $1 the United States invests in NIH, $2.56 worth of economic activity is generated (United for Medical Research, 2025). Cutting government funding for research will impede innovation, limit opportunities for private entities that rely on publicly funded research, and ultimately stall economic activity. Therefore, the report is unwavering in acknowledging that there is a strong public interest in sustaining the U.S.' position as the global leader in biomedical innovation.

REFERENCES

Austin, D., and T. Hayford, 2021. *Research and development in the pharmaceutical industry*. Washington, DC: Congressional Budget Office.

CDC (Centers for Disease Control and Prevention). 2024a. *About chronic diseases*. https://www.cdc.gov/chronic-disease/about/index.html (accessed April 2, 2025).

CDC. 2024b. *Social determinants of health*. https://www.cdc.gov/health-disparities-hiv-std-tb-hepatitis/about/social-determinants-of-health.html (accessed April 2, 2025).

CDC. 2025. *Health equity in injury and violence prevention*. https://www.cdc.gov/injury-violence-prevention/health-equity/index.html (accessed April 2, 2025).

Darrow, J. J., J. Avorn, and A. S. Kesselheim. 2020. FDA approval and regulation of pharmaceuticals, 1983-2018. *JAMA* 323(2):164–170.

Goldman, D. and D. Lakdawalla. 2018. *The global burden of medical innovation*. Brookings, January 30. https://www.brookings.edu/articles/the-global-burden-of-medical-innovation/ (accessed April 10, 2025).

Hessel, F. 2008. Burden of disease. *Encyclopedia of public health*. New York: Springer Science + Business. Pp. 94–96.

Kaitin, K. I., N. R. Phelan, D. Raiford, and B. Morris. 1991. Therapeutic ratings and end-of-phase II conferences: Initiatives to accelerate the availability of important new drugs. *Journal of Clinical Pharmacology* 31(1):17–24.

Kergall, P., E. Autin, M. Guillon, and V. Clément. 2021. Coverage and pricing recommendations of the French National Health Authority for innovative drugs: A retrospective analysis from 2014 to 2020. *Value in Health* 24(12):1784–1791.

Millum, J. 2024. Ethics and health research priority setting: A narrative review [version 1; peer review: 2 approved]. *Wellcome Open Research* 9(203).

Morgan, S. G., K. L. Bassett, J. M. Wright, R. G. Evans, M. L. Barer, P. A. Caetano, and C. D. Black. 2005. "Breakthrough" drugs and growth in expenditure on prescription drugs in Canada. *BMJ* 331(7520):815–816.

NASEM (National Academies of Sciences, Engineering, and Medicine). 2018. *Making medicines affordable: A national imperative.* Washington, DC: The National Academies Press.

NASEM. 2019. *Integrating social care into the delivery of health care: Moving upstream to improve the nation's health.* Washington, DC: The National Academies Press.

NASEM. 2022. *Improving representation in clinical trials and research: Building research equity for women and underrepresented groups.* Washington, DC: The National Academies Press.

NASEM. 2023. *Toward equitable innovation in health and medicine: A framework.* Washington, DC: The National Academies Press.

Rodwin, M. A., J. Mancini, S. Duran, A. C. Jalbert, P. Viens, D. Maraninchi, A. Gonçalves, and P. Marino. 2021. The use of "added benefit" to determine the price of new anti-cancer drugs in France, 2004–2017. *European Journal of Cancer* 145:11–18.

Sertkaya, A., T. Beleche, A. Jessup, and B. D. Sommers. 2024. Costs of drug development and research and development intensity in the U.S., 2000-2018. *JAMA Network Open* 7(6):e2415445.

United for Medical Research. 2025. *NIH's role in sustaining the U.S. economy.* https://www.unitedformedicalresearch.org/wp-content/uploads/2025/03/UMR_NIH-Role-in-Sustaining-US-Economy-FY2024-2025-Update.pdf (accessed May 28, 2025).

Wieseler, B., N. McGauran, and T. Kaiser. 2019. New drugs: Where did we go wrong and what can we do better? *BMJ* 366:l4340.

Wouters, O. J., and A. S. Kesselheim. 2024. Quantifying research and development expenditures in the drug industry. *JAMA Network Open* 7(6):e2415407.

2

Conceptual Foundations for Measuring Disease Burden, Unmet Need, and Investment in Therapeutic Development in the United States

In a 1998 report from the Institute of Medicine (IOM) titled *Scientific Opportunities and Public Needs: Improving Priority Setting and Public Input at the National Institutes of Health*, a key recommendation was for the National Institutes of Health (NIH) to "strengthen its analysis and use of health data, such as burdens and costs of disease," in determining priorities (IOM, 1998a, p.5). A study by Gross and colleagues (1999), published soon after the release of the IOM report compared NIH funding across disease areas in 1996 against several measures of disease burden, including total mortality, years of life lost, disability-adjusted life-years (DALYs), hospital days, incidence, and prevalence. The study found that funding was strongly correlated with the number of DALYs but not with the other examined metrics, and it identified specific examples of disease areas that were funded at high or low levels relative to disease burden. In addition to the Gross study, a number of other studies have used similar designs to examine the relationship between burden of disease and research funding from NIH (Carter and Gevorkian, 2025; Rees et al., 2021) and the Centers for Disease Control and Prevention (CDC) (Curry et al., 2006). These studies have commonly focused on total DALYs as the primary measure of disease burden, although some studies have included other measures such as years of life lost (Stockmann et al., 2014). Most studies have followed Gross in looking at public research funding as the comparator, though some studies have been conducted on the alignment between disease burden and funding from the pharmaceutical industry (Jung et al., 2020).

This committee was tasked to answer a question that is related in some ways to the question of alignment between research funding and burden of disease, although different in other ways. Key areas of difference include (1) a focus on therapeutic innovation rather than on all of health research; (2) a focus on unmet need for effective therapies, excluding need relating to lack of access; and (3) a broader mandate to address not only overall population burden but also burden relating to high-impact, low-frequency diseases, as well as variation in burden across different populations. Given this charge, an important foundational task is to present a clear conceptual framework for evaluating misalignment of investments in therapeutic innovations.

The committee proposes an overall rubric for identifying mismatch between investments in therapeutic innovation and disease burden or unmet need that defines underinvestment in a therapeutic area when all of the following conditions are met: (1) the therapeutic area meets one or more criteria for high disease burden; (2) the burden is insufficiently addressed by existing therapeutic options (i.e., there is an unmet need for effective therapies); and (3) the current level of investment in therapeutic development is insufficient to respond to the unmet need. For each of these conditions, this report seeks to provide a clear conceptual definition, as well as to discuss the data and measurement challenges associated with operationalizing metrics that are compatible with these conceptual definitions. This chapter focuses on the conceptual definitions and foundations. Chapter 3 will examine empirical data on areas of alignment or mismatch.

DISEASE BURDEN

Historically, public health measures for comparing the magnitude of different health problems have focused on measures of frequency, especially counts of deaths or crude population death rates. Tables of causes of death data can be traced back over several centuries, with early precedents in John Graunt's analyses of bills of mortality in London (Connor, 2024), through the development of the first classification systems for causes of death by William Farr and others (Alharbi et al., 2021). A key development in capturing a more nuanced understanding of disease burden—capturing both the event of death and the importance of its timing—is attributable to Mary Dempsey's research on tuberculosis (TB) mortality during the 1940s (Dempsey, 1947). Dempsey observed that many TB deaths occurred among younger adults and proposed that the health losses associated with tuberculosis mortality should be calculated in terms of the number of years individuals would have lived had they not died from TB. The "years of life lost" metric compared with a reference life expectancy measure became the foundation for the concept of premature mortality that has remained a central component of disease burden measurement. A number of variants of the years-of-life-lost concept followed Dempsey's precedent (CDC, 1998).

The next fundamental expansion in concepts of disease burden was the development of summary measures of population health that captured health losses related to both mortality and morbidity. Research on health-related quality of life gathered momentum in the latter part of the twentieth century, with a proliferation of quality of life measurement instruments starting in the 1960s and 1970s. The quality-adjusted life-year (QALY) was introduced in the 1970s as a summary measure for the benefits of health interventions that captured improvements in both longevity and in health-related quality of life (Spencer et al., 2022). In 1993, the disability-adjusted life-year, or DALY, was introduced as a summary measure analogous to the QALY but used to quantify and compare the population health burden associated with different causes of disease and injury (Chen et al., 2015). The first major application of DALYs to compute the global burden of disease appeared in the 1993 World Development Report (World Bank, 1993). An influential Institute of Medicine report in 1998 (IOM, 1998b) examined some of the key conceptual, empirical, and ethical issues around construction of summary measures of population health. Work at the World Health Organization during the 1990s and 2000s continued to develop frameworks and applications for use of DALYs and other summary population health measures to quantify disease burden at global and national scales (Murray et al., 2002).

In the 1990s, the World Bank commissioned the Global Burden of Disease (GBD) study to systematically estimate disability and death resulting from specific causes. The GBD study and its future iterations, while not comprehensive, are singular in their simultaneous immense scope and granularity of data (Murray, 2022). As of 2015, the Institute for Health Metrics and Evaluation (IHME), which serves as the coordinating center for GBD reports, has taken on the production of regular updates on disease burden using DALYs (IHME, n.d.).

Framework for Operationalizing the Definitions of Disease Burden

To operationalize disease burden for the purposes of the statement of task, the committee reviewed a range of previous efforts to define frameworks for the measurement of disease burden. One example is the framework published by the RTI group (Honeycutt et al., 2011), which characterizes disease burden in terms of the frequency of disease occurrences and their impact on individuals and populations. In this framework, disease occurrence is expressed by epidemiologic measures, namely, the incidence and prevalence of a disease. The committee acknowledges that the burden of a disease depends not only on how many people acquire a disease (incidence) but also on how long the people live with the disease (duration), and that the number of people currently living with a disease (prevalence) is a function of both incidence and duration. The severity of a disease, irrespective of chronicity, has a major effect on both the quality of life and economic well-being at the individual and societal levels. While important to the concept of disease burden, emerging threats, such as multidrug-resistant bacteria infections, are not covered in this chapter, though the topic is discussed in Chapter 4. To guide the task for this report, the committee adopted an operational definition of disease burden as the total, cumulative consequences of a defined disease, which in its broadest formulation includes health, social aspects, and costs to society. The measures for operationalizing this definition are discussed below.

Measures of Disease Burden on Society

Disability-Adjusted Life-Years (DALYs)

DALYs were developed as a measure of the population health effect caused by fatal and nonfatal health outcomes (Berkley et al., 1993). As such, the arithmetic components for calculating DALYs are years of life lost (YLLs) attributable to premature death and years lived with disability (YLDs) associated with nonfatal injuries and diseases. A number of critiques of DALYs have challenged key conceptual and methodological aspects of the measure as it has evolved. Early iterations of the DALY were criticized for using health experts' assessments of disability, rather than the lived experiences of people living with a disability (Grosse et al., 2009). Because of this critique, weights for nonfatal outcomes in DALYs have been based on population surveys since the 2010 iteration of the GBD study (Salomon et al., 2012). DALYs have also been criticized for devaluing the consequences in older versus younger persons that results from measuring premature mortality as a function of age at death. Furthermore, given that measures of DALYs capture the perceived desirability of health states, these measures may not be fully representative of the actual functional limitations or social participation restrictions (Grosse et al., 2009). Finally, DALYs are frequently criticized for the utilitarian nature of aggregate measures of population health as opposed to measures that include equity and distributional considerations. While some have proposed alternatives to DALYs, including the healthy life-year (Hyder et al., 1998) or narrower measures of avoidable mortality (Garcia et al., 2024; OECD, 2022) no alternative metrics have been applied with either the scope or the frequency that is found with the application of DALYs in comprehensive, standardized, and regularly updated cycles of disease burden measurement.

Quality-Adjusted Life-Years (QALYs)

The QALY measure is commonly used in the economic evaluation of health programs, medications, and technologies (Ferko et al., 2008; Touré et al., 2021). This composite measure estimates the years of life remaining for a patient following a particular treatment, medication, or technology, by weighing each year with a quality-of-life score based on multiple dimensions such as mobility, pain, and anxiety/depression. A score of *0* indicates death, while *1* indicates perfect health (Touré et al., 2021). Thus, QALYs allow for comparisons of benefits between two treatments when the outcomes and adverse effects vary (Rand and Kesselheim, 2021). There are numerous instruments available to assess QALYs (Tonin et al., 2021). Importantly, QALYs are based on average population outcomes, and as such, should be applied to treatments at a population level rather than at the individual patient level (Rand and Kesselheim, 2021). Although conceptually similar to DALYs, the QALY is not typically used as a direct measure of disease burden because it is not a standardized normative metric, so there are no comprehensive tabulations of QALYs by disease comparable to those that exist for DALYs.

The use of QALYs is controversial, with one study noting concerns that the measure is not patient focused, has the potential to be used as rationing tools by health insurers, and may be "dehumanizing" (Neumann and Cohen, 2018). Another literature review categorized criticisms of QALYs into three broad categories related to methodological issues, neutrality, and potential for discrimination (Rand and Kesselheim, 2021). Regarding methodological issues, some scholars have raised concerns about the reliability and validity among QALY instruments, the difficulty with self-reporting for some populations, and the insensitivity of the measure to specific conditions or changes in health, among other areas (Rand and Kesselheim, 2021). It is important to note that because of the instrument's weighting methods, Congress prohibited the use of QALYs in making coverage or reimbursement decisions and in pricing negotiations.[1,2] Regarding neutrality, the literature indicates that QALYs may ignore the distribution of health conditions as well as the initial severity of the conditions. The aggregation of outcomes is also a challenge with QALYs, with the measure not drawing a clear distinction between the ability to save or extend lives and improve quality of life.

Despite limitations of the metric, QALYs are often used as a unit of health benefit for intervention evaluation and cost-effectiveness analysis in the United States and worldwide. However, economists in the United

---

[1] 42 USC 1320e–1. *Limitations on certain uses of comparative clinical effectiveness research.* https://www.law.cornell.edu/uscode/text/42/1320e-1.

[2] 42 USC 1320f–3. *Negotiation and renegotiation process.* https://www.law.cornell.edu/uscode/text/42/1320f-3.

States have recently advanced alternative measures to try to account for criticisms of the QALY. For example, the equal value of life-years gained, one proposed alternative, assigns an equal value to all life-years gained and incorporates improvements in quality of life, regardless of age or disability (ICER, 2020; O'Day et al., 2021).

Health-Related Quality of Life (HRQoL)

Health-related quality-of-life (HRQoL) measures are designed to capture information on an individual's health and its effect on related areas, such as physical functioning, emotional or mental functioning, social functioning, pain, fatigue, and other symptoms (Lapin, 2020; Leininger et al., 2023). These measures have been used to inform clinical management decisions and health policy, evaluate patient outcomes, monitor patient progress and treatment response, and assess the effects of medical interventions (Lapin, 2020). A number of studies have validated the use of HRQoL across clinical and community settings, and a wide variety of validated instruments is available to assess HRQoL (Lapin, 2020; Slabaugh et al., 2017; Zack, 2013).

Typically, HRQoL measures are not used on their own as a measure of burden. Rather, they are components of summary measures like DALYs and QALYs and provide an assessment of patients' condition and functional status. Since these measures do not capture burden over time or mortality risk, they are not candidates to serve as a summary measure of disease burden, but HRQoL can provide insight into key dimensions of burden at points in time.

Despite research supporting the use of HRQoL, a number of concerns have been raised about these measures. For example, the wide range of instruments available increases the potential for inconsistent use and poor replicability by researchers (Kaplan and Hays, 2022). Additionally, patients can interpret and respond to HRQoL instruments based on their own experiences and values, thus making responses variable and challenging to interpret (Lapin, 2020). Missing data has also been identified as an issue (Lapin, 2020).

Underreporting is another challenge. In studies of HRQoL reporting within cancer clinical trials, Gupta et al. (2022) found that there was significant underreporting of HRQoL outcomes (< 50 percent) associated with U.S. Food and Drug Administration (FDA) drug approvals. Most of the trials reviewed by the authors reported HRQoL data in an ancillary paper or abstract, and at a time later than the FDA approval. Of those included in the study, 10 percent of approved drugs, based on response rates, showed improvement in HRQoL in registration trials (Gupta et al., 2022). There has also been limited reporting of HRQoL in the labels of drugs approved for rare diseases (Lanar et al., 2020).

Another issue is the potential to exclude certain populations and diseases in the available clinical literature. For example, patients who are not able to provide information or respond to the HRQoL instruments, such as those with cognitive, linguistic, or motor deficits, may be excluded from related data, resulting in selection bias and an inability to provide a representative sample of patients (Lapin, 2020). Another study assessed the validity, reliability, and responsiveness of HRQoL in over 46,000 high-cost, high-need (HCHN) adults (Leininger et al., 2023). The results indicated that an assessment of physical health exhibited robust measure validity, reliability, and responsiveness across all age groups, while the mental health scale did not (Leininger et al., 2023). The authors noted that patient-reported health outcomes remain poor in HCHN populations, even after health care usage regresses (Leininger et al., 2023).

Economic Measures of Disease Burden on Society

The metrics discussed so far are all intended to capture a construct of disease burden that relates strictly to health rather than encompassing economic outcomes. In contrast, there are proposed measures of burden that focus exclusively on these economic outcomes. These measures aim to calculate diseases' economic cost to society. It is important to recognize that society as a whole bears the cost of U.S. disease burden, through higher insurance premiums and taxes to cover health care system spending, and these costs are likely to increase without addressing unmet needs.

The most prominent of economic measure of disease burden is the cost-of-illness (COI) approach. COI studies have been undertaken since the middle of the twentieth century to quantify the economic impact of diseases on society (Cuningham, 2023). Typically these studies capture health care expenditures, lost productivity, cost of caregiving, and other direct and indirect costs of diseases. Some COI studies have focused on specific clusters of disease, such as cardiovascular disease, while others have been more general in scope. Guidelines for COI studies from NIH and the World Health Organization (WHO) have aimed to standardize methods (Honeycutt et al., 2011; WHO, 2016, 2021). However, a number of critiques of this approach have been presented, including concerns about prioritizing conditions based on their high costs rather than on their health impact, concerns about comparability across studies, and concerns about inequities in the use of economic measures that, for example, would place a greater weight on conditions that affect higher earners. In this report, the committee does not consider cost-of-illness measures as having primary relevance to its task of identifying unmet needs for therapeutic innovation.

Measures of Disease Burden on Individuals

Because measures of aggregate population-level burden reflect the combination of frequency or extent of occurrence in a population and the consequences of these occurrences, they are not well suited to identifying conditions that are particularly consequential for the individuals affected by them. The same aggregate burden could result from a common disease with a large burden per individual, or from a rarer disease with a high burden per individual. As a result, comparisons of population burden may underemphasize conditions that are relatively uncommon but responsible for substantial health losses to individuals. In the United States, a rare disease is defined as a condition affecting fewer than 200,000 (FDA, 2024). It is important to note that while these diseases are rare individually, collectively they may affect millions of Americans, and can be especially devastating—with a lengthy diagnostic odyssey, limited treatment options, and significant effects on families and caregivers. Population-level metrics can underestimate these factors and obscure areas of unmet need or disparities across populations. While these considerations are not unique to rare diseases—highly prevalent diseases such as dementia involve a high degree of individual and caregiver burden—this situation with rare diseases, some of which little has been done to characterize the underlying mechanisms of disease, needs to be balanced with disorders that affect millions of people.

Assessing individual disease burden can complement population-level information, such as the DALYs discussed above, to provide additional insight into unmet need or disparities. Individual burden can be assessed through patient-reported outcome measures (see, for example, Churruca et al., 2021) that incorporate symptom severity and quality-of-life impacts, as well as patient and caregiver perspectives. Qualitative information can offer important additional context about lived experience, challenges in diagnosis or treatment burden, effects on family and relationships, disruptions to careers and education, and more. See Box 2-1 for more discussion of patient engagement throughout the process of therapeutic development.

Variations in Disease Burden Across Different Populations

Variations in disease burden across populations have long been documented (HHS, 1985; IOM, 2003; NASEM, 2024). Disease epidemiology is known to vary in the United States across demographic attributes such as socioeconomic status, gender, age, and racial or ethnic group identity. For example, lower-income groups are at higher risk of chronic disease, including diabetes, heart disease, and chronic lung conditions (Blackwell et al., 2014; Gitterman et al., 2016; Healthy People 2030, n.d.) Associated with exposure to chronic stress, income-related health disparities are

BOX 2-1
Patient Engagement Throughout the Life
Cycle of Drug Development

To better understand how to incorporate patient voices into measures of disease burden and unmet need, the committee held a panel focused on patient engagement (see full agenda in Appendix A) during which the committee heard from patient groups and experts in patient engagement. The content in this box is based on those presentations.

Speakers highlighted several challenges in patient engagement within industry. First, speakers encouraged incorporating patient perspectives from the study outset and avoiding retroactively seeking patient perspectives, which slows down development and can result in wasted time. "Although the purpose of medicines is to improve patients' lives and to provide more effective health care, current patient involvement during medicine development and life cycle management is fragmentary at best, and mostly confined to postlaunch or late-stage clinical development" (Hoos et al., 2015, p. 930). Sometimes acquisitions occur for a promising drug where the science is there, but speakers acknowledged that it does not address an outcome that is important to the patient. Speakers also described barriers in communication, specifically that patient groups are overwhelmed with requests to replicate the same work. A proposed solution to this type of redundancy could be in the form of easily accessible repositories, such as resources from Food and Drug Administration (FDA, 2021a) and the Patient-Centered Outcomes Research Institute that could be expanded (PCORI, n.d.).

To address these challenges, Marc Boutin, the global head of patient engagement at Novartis, cited the company's Five Decision Point patient engagement framework that spans the entire life cycle of medicine development and incorporates patient insight early in therapeutic development (Patients as Partners, 2023). This framework is based on work from University of Maryland's Center of Excellence in Regulatory Science and Innovation (M-CERSI, 2025).

1. Target product profile definition: Engage patients to understand their needs and preferences to shape the desired characteristics of a new therapy.

2. Clinical trial design: Collaborate with patients to codesign trials, ensuring protocols are patient friendly and relevant.

3. Regulatory review preparation: Incorporate patient input to inform benefit–risk assessments during regulatory submissions.

continued

BOX 2-1 Continued

4. Market access strategy: Engage patients to inform pricing, reimbursement, and access strategies, facilitating equitable access.

5. Postmarket activities: Involve patients in real-world effectiveness monitoring and gathering feedback for continuous improvement.

By engaging patients at the beginning of research through clinical development, Boutin cited faster drug development times that cut as much as 2.5–3.5 months off the clinical development timeline. In addition to saved time, early and consistent patient engagement generated $250 million in savings for the company and created a net present value between $850 million and $1.5 billion.

SOURCE: Panelists' remarks to the committee in public session on December 16, 2024.

---

documented across the life course. In particular, experiencing childhood poverty is associated with nutritional deficits, developmental delays, and other adverse health outcomes in the long term (Gitterman et al., 2016; Pascoe et al., 2016). Poverty contributes to higher mortality and lower life expectancy for those with lower incomes (Healthy People 2030, n.d.; Khullar and Chokshi, 2018). In addition to health consequences, people with lower incomes face barriers to accessing health care or paying for treatments (Healthy People 2030, n.d.; Khullar and Chokshi, 2018).

In another example of varied disease burden, rural populations tend to have higher rates of smoking (and associated chronic illnesses), high blood pressure, obesity, and unintentional injury deaths (CDC, 2024a); these risks are compounded by less accessible health care and lower health care usage (Nuako et al., 2022). Conversely, urban populations are at higher risk of exposure to air pollution, but this exposure is differentially distributed—lower income, Hispanic, and Black populations are more likely to live in urban areas with high levels of pollutants and are thus more at risk for negative health impacts (American Lung Association, 2023; Kerr et al., 2024).

Similarly, disease burden and health outcomes often vary across racial and ethnic groups, typically caused by differential exposure to positive and negative social determinants of health or other factors associated with race and ethnicity, rather than any inherent biological difference. For instance, maternal mortality rates are highly disproportionate, with pregnant women who identify as Black, American Indian or Alaska Native, or Native Hawaiian or Pacific Islander being over three times more likely than White individuals to experience a pregnancy-related death (CDC, 2024b; Hill et al., 2024). In another recent report, American Indians and Alaska Natives have the lowest average estimated life expectancy at birth compared to other racial and ethnic groups in the United States (Arias et al., 2023). There are numerous other examples of variations in disease burden across populations (see NASEM, 2024).

In sum, health disparities can stem from a variety of factors including historical context, environmental exposures, and social determinants of health. These variations in disease burden can illuminate different areas of unmet need where innovation could help close gaps. For example, innovative point-of-care diagnostics and treatments could make higher-quality care more accessible for rural populations who reside far from urban medical centers.

The Effect of Comorbidities

In evaluating the burden of individual diseases, it is important to consider not just the burden directly related to the disease itself, but also the potential for one disease to increase the risk of developing additional comorbid diseases or to adversely affect the course of existing comorbid disease(s). Multimorbidity, defined as two or more coexisting conditions, affects 58.4 percent of adults in the United States (Mossadeghi et al., 2023). The prevalence of multimorbidity increases with age but affects people across all age spectra; among those aged 20–29 years, the prevalence is 22.2 percent (Mossadeghi et al., 2023).

Failure to consider the effect of individual diseases on the occurrence or course of comorbid diseases and related downstream health-related expenditures could result in substantial undervaluations or, less commonly, overvaluations of the burden for a given disease. Among people with multiple comorbid chronic diseases, overall spending on health care was multiplicative, meaning that spending for the combination of diseases was significantly higher than for the diseases individually, for more than 60 percent of the U.S. population (Chang et al., 2023).

Major depressive disorder provides an instructive example of how one disease can increase the risk of developing other diseases, adversely affect the course of existing comorbid diseases, and thereby increase downstream health-related expenditures (Box 2-2).

Beyond depression, several other mental health disorders are associated with an increased risk for a range of medical conditions (Rapsey et al., 2015; Scott et al., 2016). A population-based cohort study of nearly

BOX 2-2
Exemplar: Major Depressive Disorder

Major depressive disorder (MDD) is considerably more common in people with common general medical conditions than it is in people without them (Walker et al., 2018; Wang et al., 2017). While the prevalence of MDD is approximately 5 percent in the general population (GBD 2016 Disease and Injury Incidence and Prevalence Collaborators, 2017), its prevalence is substantially higher among adults with type 2 diabetes (28 percent) (Khaledi et al., 2019), myocardial infarction (29 percent) (Doyle et al., 2015), cerebrovascular disease (~18 percent) (Mitchell et al., 2017), or cancer (8–24 percent) (Krebber et al., 2014).

A recent large (n = 130,652) multicohort study of UK Biobank participants highlights the contribution of depression to excess hospitalizations for a range of medical conditions (Frank et al., 2023). In a series of adjusted Cox proportional hazards regressions, severe or moderately severe depression was associated with increased hazards-of-incident hospital admissions for multiple conditions, including bacterial infections and ischemic heart disease. There is also evidence that depression accelerates the progression of comorbid diseases. Among participants in the UK Biobank study with prevalent heart conditions, those with depression at baseline had nearly twice the risk of hospital admission for circulatory conditions during follow-up as those without depression at baseline (Frank et al., 2023).

Several mechanisms may account for why individuals with depression are at increased risk for these and other diseases. For example, the elevated rates of obesity (de Wit et al., 2010) and diminished physical activity (Schuch et al., 2017) seen among adults with depression could contribute to their elevated risk of developing type 2 diabetes (Yu et al., 2015), stroke (Pan et al., 2011), or coronary artery disease (Cao et al., 2022). Of course, the co-occurrence of depression with these and other medical conditions might also be confounded by earlier exposures to childhood abuse, socioeconomic adversities, substance use, or shared environmental or genetic risk factors. A review identified 24 candidate genes that are shared between depression and cardiovascular disease (Amare et al., 2017). For these reasons, attributing to depression all the excess increased risk burden of comorbid medical conditions observed in these epidemiological studies risks overestimating the global disease burden of depression.

A similar challenge exists in deciding what fraction of the increased burden associated with accelerated comorbid disease progression to assign to depression. It is possible that by reducing adherence to treatment (Gold et al., 2020) or diminishing aspects of self-care (Morgan et al., 2006), depression tends to accelerate the progression of several chronic preexisting diseases. Again, however, shared environmental and genetic factors may contribute to the liability to develop depression and to a poorer course of comorbid medical conditions.

6 million individuals from Danish registries revealed that in addition to mood disorders, there are strong prospective associations of substance-use disorders, anxiety disorders, schizophrenia, eating disorders, personality disorders, intellectual disabilities, developmental disorders, behavioral disorders, and organic disorders with many general medical conditions (Momen et al., 2020). Research indicates that the burden of mental health disorders is manifested not only through direct effects on health care and health care costs, reduced productivity, and diminished quality of life, but also indirectly through increased risks of developing other general medical conditions and accelerated progression of comorbid medical conditions. Because mental health disorders commonly have adverse effects on health behaviors including self-care, it is not surprising that many mental health disorders are associated with an increased risk of developing general medical conditions and poorer outcomes of existing persistent medical conditions.

The possibility of bidirectional associations between two diseases complicates the attribution of disease burden to a single disease. For example, individuals with rheumatoid arthritis are at increased risk of developing depression, while those with depression are also at increased risk of developing rheumatoid arthritis (Lu et al., 2016). The mechanisms underlying these connections are incompletely understood. However, they might involve rheumatoid arthritis-mediated physical limitations and work restrictions for the former association, and depression-mediated dysregulation of the hypothalamic–pituitary adrenal axis related expression of inflammatory cytokines for the latter.

In addition to mental health conditions, there are also many important examples of general medical conditions being strong risk factors for related medical conditions. A few well-known examples include hypertension and cardiovascular disease (including stroke, peripheral arterial disease, coronary artery disease, renal disease, heart failure, atrial fibrillation) (Alloubani et al., 2018; Glovaci et al., 2019), ulcerative colitis and colorectal cancer (Lakatos and Lakatos, 2008), and peptic ulcer disease with gastric cancer (Hansson et al., 1996).

The effect of diabetes mellitus highlights how one condition can affect downstream outcomes for unmet needs. Diabetes affects 38.4 million people in the United States., which represents more than 11 percent of the entire population (NIDDK, 2024). Of these, 352,000 are children and adolescents under the age of 20.

It is well established that diabetes leads to microvascular complications: retinopathy (diabetes is the leading cause of blindness), neuropathy, and nephropathy/kidney disease (Klein, 1995). Additionally, diabetes leads to macrovascular complications, including coronary artery disease, peripheral arterial disease, and cerebrovascular disease (Arnold et al., 2022). These risks include those of acute myocardial infarction (Sarnak et al., 2019) and stroke (Kaze et al., 2022). Furthermore, there is an additive effect of the microvascular complications on the macrovascular complications; for example, kidney disease among people with diabetes also independently increases the risk of acute myocardial infarction and stroke. Therefore, diabetes leads to additional comorbidities and these comorbidities also lead to adverse downstream health outcomes for patients. As another example of these complex relationships, one of the strongest recommendations for patients who develop these macrovascular complications is physical activity (which is well established to reduce the risk of acute myocardial infarction and stroke). However, patients with diabetes, who are at much higher risk of developing neuropathy, may then be limited in their ability to perform physical activity—including walking (Kanade et al., 2006).

This cascade of comorbidities and sequelae of diabetes also increases health care spending beyond just care for diabetes. It is estimated that the total cost of diagnosed diabetes in the United States in 2022 was $412.9 billion (Parker et al., 2024). Attributable primarily to the vascular complications of diabetes, the mean annual all-cause costs for people with type 2 diabetes were nearly 2.6 times higher than control patients without diabetes in the year after diagnosis and stabilized to between 1.5 and 1.6 times higher in the 2 to 8 years postdiagnosis (Visaria et al., 2020).

In summary, the occurrence of one disorder commonly increases the risk of developing other disorders or adversely affecting the progression of comorbid disorders. The interlinked nature of disease processes poses a critical challenge to the accurate attribution of societal burden and spending on specific individual diseases. Investing in research to help dissect the complex causal pathways linking diseases to each other and to their progression will not only improve the targeting of preventive interventions but also improve the precision with which disease-specific burdens are estimated.

The Committee's Approach to Assessing Disease Burden

In summary, these measures of disease burden all feature some measurements of the epidemiology, economic impact, and health-related quality of life of diseases. Given the multiple existing measures of disease burden, the committee did not create new measures but rather sought to use existing measures and data to help address and accomplish the statement of task. Moreover, considering the variety of ways that disease burden can be measured and analyzed, the committee recognized that there was no single method for assessing mismatch. As covered in this section, all quantitative measures of disease burden or health gains have a degree of subjectivity because they incorporate different assumptions or ethical judgments. Different approaches used to address disease burden could also stem from different priorities and hence yield varied results. Thus, the committee does not propose a single metric or approach for determining mismatch between burden and investment, but instead considers applying several dimensions and factors, such as both population-level and individual burden, that would inform mismatch or alignment. Any prioritization system involves some kind of value judgments and trade-offs, but having clear and transparent metrics is important to move beyond the current system.

To improve the assessment of disease burden for the purposes of investment decisions, it is important to align on standardized disease and therapeutic categories for comparison. Similarly, given the long development time of therapeutics, informative assessments of disease burden will need to incorporate estimates of future burden. For instance, such estimates will be particularly useful in better understanding how climate-induced changes in the distribution of vector-borne infectious diseases will affect U.S. disease burden. Forecast scenarios will also reflect the steady evolution of demographic (e.g., life expectancy) and epidemiological (e.g., risk factors) changes that have been well characterized in previous retrospective analyses, such as the GBD decomposition analyses (GBD, 2024), as well as other drivers that are less predictable but could have important implications for unmet need. For example, future estimates are also necessary to account for the risk of low-probability, high-impact events, such as pandemics and natural disasters, even if their low probabilities make them inherently hard to predict.

In the following chapter, the committee analyzes available data to assess mismatch, to the extent possible given some data limitations (see Chapter 3).

UNMET NEED

Unmet need refers to treatment gaps or areas where therapies do not exist for a particular medical condition or existing therapies are either inadequate or inaccessible (Lodato and Kaplan, 2013). In cases where there are existing therapies, unmet need may arise in relation to limitations in efficacy, safety, tolerability, convenience, or accessibility. A focus on unmet need highlights the medical areas where improved treatment options are needed to more effectively address patient health concerns (Vreman et al., 2019).

Unmet need exists when a patient population lacks adequate therapeutic interventions to effectively manage or cure a condition. This definition centers on the needs of patients and helps identify areas of therapeutic development to prioritize in order to address these unmet needs and to improve associated disease burden. FDA guidance similarly defines unmet medical need as "a condition whose treatment or diagnosis is not addressed adequately by available therapy" (FDA, 2014, p. 4). If approved therapies exist, new treatments could still address FDA's definition of unmet medical need under several conditions such as having an improved effect on a serious health outcome, improving outcomes in patients who did not respond to available therapy, and reducing the potential for harmful drug interactions or side effects, among others (FDA, 2014).

To summarize this discussion and to define the scope of this report, the committee considered a continuum of unmet need (Figure 2-1), recognizing that this is a generalization that does not capture the nuances of what drives unmet need. (See Chapter 4 for a discussion of factors that contribute to misalignment between innovation, disease burden, and unmet need.) On one end of the spectrum is "no effective treatment"—that is, there are no currently approved therapeutic treatment options for a particular disease condition. At the other end of the spectrum are conditions with effective and accessible treatments. Between these points is a range of conditions for which treatments have limited effectiveness or low tolerability. As the examples discussed in this section demonstrate, existing treatments may be associated with residual unmet need for a variety of reasons (e.g., low tolerability, difficulty managing treatment regimens, insufficient improvements to health outcomes). In this framework, effectiveness is considered a composite of efficacy and tolerability that represents not only how well a treatment works under ideal conditions (efficacy) but also how well it is tolerated by patients (tolerability) under real-world conditions.

Limited access to or use of existing therapeutics, in general or for subgroups of the population, can also contribute to unmet need, though as noted in Chapter 1, considerations for individual access are considered out of scope for this report. Some dimensions of access are inseparable from notions of unmet need relevant to innovation priorities, including features of the technology itself, the clinical context in which it is used, and the current drug pricing and reimbursement system. These dimensions are discussed more fully in the chapters that follow.

Level of unmet need

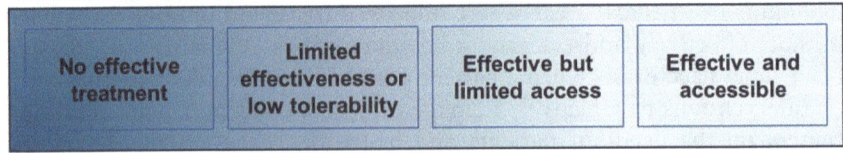

FIGURE 2-1 Categorization of unmet need.
NOTE: The committee considered a continuum of unmet need, categorized as a medical condition or disease for which there are (1) no existing effective therapeutic treatment options, (2) existing therapeutic solutions with limited effectiveness, or (3) existing effective and tolerable therapies that have limited access.

However, this report will not consider in detail the broader social, economic, and behavioral determinants that influence patient access and use of existing treatments. Such determinants include disparities in our health care system overall that lead to underdiagnosis and inadequate treatment, economic barriers associated with out-of-pocket costs of the drugs and associated follow-on care, disparities in education and health literacy that lead to substandard care receipt, and the neighborhood and built environment, which can limit access to preventive services and health promoting behaviors. A better understanding of how these determinants and others affect access to and use of existing therapeutics will be critical if there is to be a significant reduction in unmet need, but these themes are beyond the scope of this report.

Factors That Contribute to Unmet Need

The committee recognizes that it is challenging to develop a uniform understanding of what areas constitute an unmet need given the many factors that can contribute to it. Major depressive disorder or schizophrenia, for example, each have a large number of FDA-approved pharmacological treatments, but these medications yield only modest reductions in symptoms and functional improvement (Ormel et al., 2022). In the case of schizophrenia, the most widely used medications commonly result in adverse metabolic effects contributing to substantial unmet need for safer options (Chang et al., 2021). In other conditions, therapeutic effectiveness may be limited to certain subgroups of the population based on the severity of disease presentations, subtypes of disease, or treatment resistance. With hypercholesterolemia, for instance, statins are highly effective in lowering lipid levels in a large segment of the population (Feingold, 2024). However, a significant percentage of hyperlipidemic patients, including those with familial hypercholesterolemia, are unable to reach their LDL-goals, despite adherence to statin medications (Feingold, 2024).

When innovative PCSK9 inhibitors gained FDA approval, which are effective for familial hypercholesterolemia, payer coverage was limited, given the lack of cost-effectiveness research available at the time of launch, which narrowed access to individuals who could not achieve lipid goals on statins, thereby contributing to unmet clinical need for others who may experience greater benefit from PCSK9 compared to statins (Baum et al., 2017). The time course of disease can also limit the effectiveness of available therapeutics. For instance, antiparasitic agents, such as praziquantel and metronidazole, which are indicated in neglected tropical diseases, such as schistosomiasis and amebiasis, respectively, are effective only initially, before the parasites develop resistance or tolerance, which makes them ineffective over the long term (Eastham et al., 2024; Shrivastav et al., 2021).

Unfavorable safety profiles and low tolerability can also limit the ability of existing therapeutics to address disease burden and can result in residual unmet need. Treatment of idiopathic pulmonary fibrosis (IPF) offers an example. Nintedanib (OFEV) and pirfenidone (Esbriet) are associated with significant adverse effects yet remain the primary antifibrotic options for idiopathic pulmonary fibrosis, which is a condition with a high associated mortality (He et al., 2024). A next generation of pirfenidone, a deuterated analogue, recently passed FDA phase 2 clinical trials with an improved safety and tolerability profile (Waldron, 2024). While not entirely novel, these improvements demonstrate innovation and may make the drug better suited to the IPF patient population, potentially helping to reduce unmet need.

Available therapies may also not be able to address unmet need because of problems related to clinical distribution, use, and adherence. Patients with schizophrenia, for instance, who may not be aware of their need for treatment, often present with limited adherence to treatment regimens, which prevents them from benefiting from antipsychotic agents (Olfson et al., 2006). As another example, medications that require refrigeration or cold-chain management may be limited in addressing disease burden in underserved areas that lack the infrastructure to support cold-chain requirements or for people who lack stable housing (Deloitte, 2023; IOM, 1988). Finally, the committee recognizes that unmet need may result not only from lack of effective treatment options, but in some cases from lack of accurate diagnostics that enable timely and precise identification of treatment need, as well as accurate predictive information on patients who are most likely to respond to a specific treatment.

An illustrative example of how unmet need reflects more than simply the availability of efficacious therapies, and how it relates to access and adherence, is the persistent burden of HIV infection in the United States and globally despite the development of highly effective preexposure prophylaxis (PrEP). In 2012, the first PrEP medication was approved by FDA (Gilead, 2012). A major advance was made in 2021 with the introduction of a long-acting injectable PrEP (FDA, 2021b). While both forms of administration have been shown to be over 99 percent effective in reducing infection when taken as prescribed, one study showed that, in practice, the risk of HIV infection was 66 percent lower among those using the injectable versus oral PrEP; the difference was largely attributable to lower adherence to the oral (once a day) regimen versus the long-acting injectable drug, which is administered once every 2 months (Landovitz et al., 2021). Other formulation and delivery options are being tested and show promise, including HIV self-testing-supported models of oral PrEP delivery that rely on self-testing and can reduce the number of needed clinical visits (Kiptinness et al., 2022). The contrast in effectiveness between the two different forms of PrEP illustrates well how unmet need may persist even when effective therapies are available, and technological innovation to reduce unmet need can do so by addressing barriers to access and adherence.

Yet despite the availability of multiple PrEP options, fewer than one-quarter of the estimated 1.2 million people in the United States who could benefit from PrEP receive prescriptions (Powder, 2022). Once PrEP is prescribed, adherence can be low or not sustained over long periods of time, especially with the oral PrEP (Ó Murchu et al., 2022). Barriers to both access and adherence include lack of awareness of one's risk and how PrEP can help reduce that risk, HIV-related stigma, access to health care providers who are knowledgeable about the benefits of PrEP, high costs and inadequate insurance coverage, and perceived concerns about side effects which include headaches, fatigue, and gastric pain, but are usually mild and transitory. As one review concluded: "The future of PrEP adherence lies in person-centered approaches to service delivery that meet the needs of individuals while creating supportive environments and facilitating health-care access and delivery" (Haberer et al., 2023, p. 1).

In summary, unmet need comprises a lack of available treatments and deficiencies in available treatments. In contrast, disease burden encompasses the overall impact of a medical condition on patient populations and society. Both unmet need and disease burden are important concepts for understanding the gaps in health care and developing innovative solutions to improve outcomes.

INVESTMENT IN THERAPEUTIC INNOVATION

The public and private sectors play complementary roles in supporting and conducting biomedical research and development (R&D) in the United States. The public sector, through federal agencies such as the NIH and the Department of Defense, is the largest funder of basic research,[3] and the private sector primarily supports and engages in drug discovery and development activities, such as clinical testing, incremental innovation (Barbosu, 2025), and product differentiation—activities that largely follow from basic research (Congressional Budget Office, 2021; Simoens and Huys, 2022).

Public investment in basic and applied biomedical research has contributed significantly to the development of new drugs (Galkina Cleary et al., 2018, 2023). As one study notes, public-sector researchers have "performed the upstream, basic research that elucidated the underlying mechanisms of disease and identified promising points of intervention"

---

[3] Basic research, also sometimes called basic science or pure research, is a type of research that seeks to uncover and understand fundamental mechanisms and phenomena—for example, about health and disease. This work typically informs more applied research.

(Stevens et al., 2011, p. 535). When one accounts for indirect support such as basic science research on drug targets, NIH funded projects related to every new FDA-approved drug from 2010 to 2016 (Galkina Cleary et al., 2018). Moreover, although the public sector is known to predominantly invest in basic research, one study showed that one in four new drugs had some later-stage research contribution (usually related to the drug's initial discovery or synthesis, and not always financial) from institutions such as universities that rely heavily on public support or from start-ups spun out of these publicly supported research institutions (Nayak et al., 2019). Public funding is less likely to directly support patentable aspects of new drugs; for example, fewer than 10 percent of drugs approved from 1985 to 2022 had any patents based on federal funding (Ouellette and Sampat, 2024). But public-sector investment has been shown to generate and amplify additional private-sector investment in biomedical research. For example, one study found that rather than "crowding out" private investment, each $10 million increase in NIH funding leads to 2.3 additional private-sector patents (Azoulay et al., 2019).

In addition to federal agencies, public-sector contributors to biomedical R&D include universities, international organizations, charities, and crowd-funding, while private-sector entities include venture capital funds, pharmaceutical and biotechnology companies, private foundations and nonprofit organizations, and private research centers (Simoens and Huys, 2022). In 2020, funding for medical and health R&D investments in the United States came from the following entities (Research!America, 2022):

- 66 percent from industry;[4]
- 25.1 percent from federal government;
- 6.9 percent from academic and research institutions;
- 1.2 percent from foundations, voluntary health associations, and professional societies; and
- 0.9 percent from state governments.

Private-sector investment in R&D can come from a variety of sources, including in-house asset development at established biopharmaceutical companies, company mergers and acquisitions, and venture capital firms (SiRM et al., 2022). For-profit private-sector funding for biopharmaceutical research is driven largely by a return-on-investment analysis, determined by the amount of expected revenue, cost, and policies influencing its development (Congressional Budget Office, 2021). Decisions about new drugs are generally made within a set of three different contexts: scientific opportunity,

---

[4] These investments do not include funding directed toward industry from other sources (Research!America, 2022).

market assessment (including medical need), and available and required resources. As private investment requires a return on investment within a predetermined time and a well-understood risk profile, some strategies and assessment for investment are centered on decreasing the timeline of R&D, decreasing the risk intrinsic in the discovery and development of new effective drugs, and increasing the willingness to pay from target payers and/or populations.

Not all private-sector R&D investment is motivated by return on investment. Private nonprofit organizations, including those that focus on specific disease areas, also fund biomedical R&D in support of their individual missions. These investments can be critical for advancing research to a stage where for-profit investors begin to see opportunities for commercialization (Graddy-Reed, 2020).

The public and private sectors are both critical for advancing drug innovation in the United States. Public investments help understand disease mechanisms that contribute to important novel drug targets and innovations from the private sector that can help reduce unmet needs.

REFERENCES

Alharbi, M. A., G. Isouard, and B. Tolchard. 2021. Historical development of the statistical classification of causes of death and diseases. *Cogent Medicine* 8(1):1893422.

Alloubani, A., A. Saleh, and I. Abdelhafiz. 2018. Hypertension and diabetes mellitus as a predictive risk factors for stroke. *Diabetes & Metabolic Syndrome* 12(4):577–584.

Amare, A. T., K. O. Schubert, M. Klingler-Hoffmann, S. Cohen-Woods, and B. T. Baune. 2017. The genetic overlap between mood disorders and cardiometabolic diseases: A systematic review of genome wide and candidate gene studies. *Translational Psychiatry* 7(1):e1007.

American Lung Association. 2023. *Disparities in the impact of air pollution.* https://www.lung.org/clean-air/outdoors/who-is-at-risk/disparities (accessed February 19, 2025).

Arias, E., J. Xu, and K. Kochanek. 2023. United States life tables, 2021. *National Vital Statistics Report* 72(12):1–64.

Arnold, S. V., K. Khunti, F. Tang, H. Chen, J. Cid-Ruzafa, A. Cooper, P. Fenici, M. B. Gomes, N. Hammar, L. Ji, G. L. Saraiva, J. Medina, A. Nicolucci, L. Ramirez, W. Rathmann, M. V. Shestakova, I. Shimomura, F. Surmont, J. Vora, H. Watada, and M. Kosiborod. 2022. Incidence rates and predictors of microvascular and macrovascular complications in patients with type 2 diabetes: Results from the longitudinal global DISCOVER study. *American Heart Journal* 243:232–239.

Azoulay, P., J. S. Graff Zivin, D. Li, and B. N. Sampat. 2019. Public R&D investments and private-sector patenting: Evidence from NIH funding rules. *Review of Economic Studies* 86(1):117–152.

Barbosu, S. 2025. *The value of follow-on biopharma innovation for health outcomes and economic growth.* Information Technology & Innovation Foundation. https://www2.itif.org/2025-follow-on-biopharma.pdf (accessed April 12, 2025).

Baum, S. J., P. P. Toth, J. A. Underberg, P. Jellinger, J. Ross, and K. Wilemon. 2017. PCSK9 inhibitor access barriers-issues and recommendations: Improving the access process for patients, clinicians and payers. *Clinical Cardiology* 40(4):243–254.

Berkley, S., J. L. Bobadilla, R. M. Hecht, K. Hill, D. T. Jamison, C. J. L. Murray, P. A. Musgrove, H. Saxenian, and J.-P. Tan. 1993. *World development report 1993: Investing in health.* Washington, DC: World Bank Group.

Blackwell, D. L., J. W. Lucas, and T. C. Clarke. 2014. Summary health statistics for U.S. adults: National Health Interview Survey, 2012. *Vital Health Statistics* 10(260):1–161.

Cao, H., H. Zhao, and L. Shen. 2022. Depression increased risk of coronary heart disease: A meta-analysis of prospective cohort studies. *Frontiers in Cardiovascular Medicine* 9. https://doi.org/10.3389/fcvm.2022.913888.

Carter, A. J. R., and M. Gevorkian. 2025. The persistence of very low correlations between NIH research funding and disease burdens. *Public Health in Practice* 9:100580.

CDC (Centers for Disease Control and Prevention). 1998. *Mortality Weekly Report Supplements.* https://www.cdc.gov/mmwr/preview/mmwrhtml/00001773.htm#:~:text=In%20 1947%2C%20as%20a%20supplement,remaining%20at%20death%20 (accessed January 23, 2025).

CDC. 2024a. *About rural health.* https://www.cdc.gov/rural-health/php/about/index.html (accessed February 19, 2025).

CDC. 2024b. *Pregnancy mortality surveillance system.* https://www.cdc.gov/reproductivehealth/ maternal-mortality/pregnancy-mortality-surveillance-system.htm (accessed February 19, 2025).

Chang, A. Y., D. Bryazka, and J. L. Dieleman. 2023. Estimating health spending associated with chronic multimorbidity in 2018: An observational study among adults in the United States. *PLoS Medicine* 20(4):e1004205.

Chang, S. C., K. K. Goh, and M. L. Lu. 2021. Metabolic disturbances associated with antipsychotic drug treatment in patients with schizophrenia: State-of-the-art and future perspectives. *World Journal of Psychiatry* 11(10):696–710.

Chen, A., K. H. Jacobsen, A. A. Deshmukh, and S. B. Cantor. 2015. The evolution of the disability-adjusted life year (DALY). *Socio-Economic Planning Sciences* 49(1):10–15.

Churruca, K., C. Pomare, L. A. Ellis, J. C. Long, S. B. Henderson, L. E. D. Murphy, C. J. Leahy, and J. Braithwaite. 2021. Patient-reported outcome measures (PROMS): A review of generic and condition-specific measures and a discussion of trends and issues. *Health Expectations* 24(4):1015–1024.

Congressional Budget Office. 2021. *Research and development in the pharmaceutical industry.* https://www.cbo.gov/publication/57126 (accessed April 12, 2025).

Connor, H. 2024. John Graunt F.R.S. (1620-74): The founding father of human demography, epidemiology and vital statistics. *Journal of Medical Biography* 32(1):57–69.

Cuningham, W. G. G. 2023. *Innovative approaches to surveillance and quantifying the burden of bacterial infections and antibiotic resistance in northern Australia.* Ph.D diss. Charles Darwin University, Australia.

Curry, C. W., A. K. De, R. M. Ikeda, and S. B. Thacker. 2006. Health burden and funding at the Centers for Disease Control and Prevention. *American Journal of Preventive Medicine* 30(3):269–276.

de Wit, L., F. Luppino, A. van Straten, B. Penninx, F. Zitman, and P. Cuijpers. 2010. Depression and obesity: A meta-analysis of community-based studies. *Psychiatry Research* 178(2):230–235.

Deloitte. 2023. *Access to medicine: Reach more patients through a deeper understanding of access issues.* https://www.deloitte.com/fr/fr/Industries/life-sciences-health-care/analysis/ access-medicine.html (accessed May 20, 2025).

Dempsey, M. 1947. Decline in tuberculosis. *American Review of Tuberculosis* 56(2):157–164.

Doyle, F., H. McGee, R. Conroy, H. J. Conradi, A. Meijer, R. Steeds, H. Sato, D. E. Stewart, K. Parakh, R. Carney, K. Freedland, M. Anselmino, R. Pelletier, E. H. Bos, and P. de Jonge. 2015. Systematic review and individual patient data meta-analysis of sex differences in depression and prognosis in persons with myocardial infarction: A mindmaps study. *Psychosomatic Medicine* 77(4):419–428.

Eastham, G., D. Fausnacht, M. H. Becker, A. Gillen, and W. Moore. 2024. Praziquantel resistance in schistosomes: A brief report. *Frontiers in Parasitology* 3.

FDA (Food and Drug Administration). 2014. *Guidance for industry expedited programs for serious conditions—drugs and biologics.* Silver Spring, MD: Food and Drug Administration. https://www.fda.gov/files/drugs/published/Expedited-Programs-for-Serious-Conditions-Drugs-and-Biologics.pdf (accessed April 12, 2025).

FDA. 2021a. *Clinical outcome assessment compendium.* https://www.fda.gov/drugs/development-resources/clinical-outcome-assessment-compendium (accessed March 19, 2025).

FDA. 2021b. *FDA approves first injectable treatment for HIV pre-exposure prevention.* https://www.fda.gov/news-events/press-announcements/fda-approves-first-injectable-treatment-hiv-pre-exposure-prevention (accessed May 21, 2025).

FDA. 2024. *Rare diseases at the FDA.* https://www.fda.gov/patients/rare-diseases-fda (accessed March 20, 2025).

Feingold, K. R. 2024. *Cholesterol lowering drugs.* https://www.ncbi.nlm.nih.gov/books/NBK395573/ (accessed May 19, 2025).

Ferko, N., M. Postma, S. Gallivan, D. Kruzikas, and M. Drummond. 2008. Evolution of the health economics of cervical cancer vaccination. *Vaccine* 26:F3–F15.

Frank, P., G. D. Batty, J. Pentti, M. Jokela, L. Poole, J. Ervasti, J. Vahtera, G. Lewis, A. Steptoe, and M. Kivimäki. 2023. Association between depression and physical conditions requiring hospitalization. *JAMA Psychiatry* 80(7):690.

Galkina Cleary, E., J. M. Beierlein, N. S. Khanuja, L. M. McNamee, and F. D. Ledley. 2018. Contribution of NIH funding to new drug approvals 2010–2016. *Proceedings of the National Academies of Sciences* 115(10):2329–2334.

Galkina Cleary, E., M. J. Jackson, E. W. Zhou, and F. D. Ledley. 2023. Comparison of research spending on new drug approvals by the National Institutes of Health vs. the pharmaceutical industry, 2010–2019. *JAMA Health Forum* 4(4):e230511.

García, M. C., L. M. Rossen, K. Matthews, G. Guy, K. F. Trivers, C. C. Thomas, L. Schieb, and M. F. Iademarco. 2024. Preventable premature deaths from the five leading causes of death in nonmetropolitan and metropolitan counties, United States, 2010–2022. *Morbidity and Mortality Weekly Report* 73:1–11.

GBD (Global Burden of Death study). 2024. Global burden of 288 causes of death and life expectancy decomposition in 204 countries and territories and 811 subnational locations: A systematic analysis for the Global Burden of Disease study 2021. *Lancet* 403(10440):2100–2132.

GBD 2016 Disease and Injury Incidence and Prevalence Collaborators. 2017. Global, regional, and national incidence, prevalence, and years lived with disability for 328 diseases and injuries for 195 countries, 1990; 2016: A systematic analysis for the Global Burden of Disease Study 2016. *Lancet* 390(10100):1211–1259.

Gilead. 2012. *U.S. Food and Drug Administration approves Gilead's Truvada for reducing the risk of acquiring HIV.* https://www.gilead.com/news/news-details/2012/us-food-and-drug-administration-approves-gileads-truvada-for-reducing-the-risk-of-acquiring-hiv#:~:text=Truvada%20for%20a%20PrEP%20indication: (accessed May 21, 2025).

Gitterman, B. A., P. J. Flanagan, W. H. Cotton, K. J. Dilley, J. H. Duffee, A. E. Green, V. A. Keane, S. D. Krugman, J. M. Linton, C. D. McKelvey, and J. L. Nelson. 2016. Poverty and child health in the United States. *Pediatrics* 137(4):e20160339.

Glovaci, D., W. Fan, and N. D. Wong. 2019. Epidemiology of diabetes mellitus and cardio-vascular disease. *Current Cardiology Reports* 21(4):21.

Gold, S. M., O. Köhler-Forsberg, R. Moss-Morris, A. Mehnert, J. J. Miranda, M. Bullinger, A. Steptoe, M. A. Whooley, and C. Otte. 2020. Comorbid depression in medical diseases. *Nature Reviews* Disease Primers 6(1):69.

Graddy-Reed, A. 2020. Getting ahead in the race for a cure: How nonprofits are financing biomedical R&D. *Research Policy* 49(8):104032.

Gross, C. P., G. F. Anderson, and N. R. Powe. 1999. The relation between funding by the National Institutes of Health and the burden of disease. *New England Journal of Medicine* 340(24):1881–1887.

Grosse, S. D., D. J. Lollar, V. A. Campbell, and M. Chamie. 2009. Disability and disability-adjusted life years: Not the same. *Public Health Reports* 124(2):197–202.

Gupta, M., O. S. Akhtar, B. Bahl, A. Mier-Hicks, K. Attwood, K. Catalfamo, B. Gyawali, and P. Torka. 2022. Is health-related quality of life (HRQoL) reporting keeping pace with new drug approvals in hematology and oncology: A five-year analysis of 245 drug approvals. *Journal of Clinical Oncology* 40(16Suppl):6519.

Haberer, J. E., A. Mujugira, and K. H. Mayer. 2023. The future of HIV pre-exposure pro-phylaxis adherence: Reducing barriers and increasing opportunities. *Lancet HIV* 10(6):e404–e411.

Hansson, L.-E., O. Nyrén, A. W. Hsing, R. Bergström, S. Josefsson, W.-H. Chow, J. F. Fraumeni, and H.-O. Adami. 1996. The risk of stomach cancer in patients with gastric or duodenal ulcer disease. *New England Journal of Medicine* 335(4):242–249.

He, M., T. Yang, J. Zhou, R. Wang, and X. Li. 2024. A real-world study of antifibrotic drugs-related adverse events based on the United States Food and Drug Administration adverse event reporting system and vigiaccess databases. *Frontiers in Pharmacology* 15.

Healthy People 2030. n.d. *Poverty*. https://odphp.health.gov/healthypeople/priority-areas/social-determinants-health/literature-summaries/poverty (accessed February 19, 2025).

HHS (Department of Health and Human Services). 1985. *Report of the Secretary's Task Force on Black & Minority Health.* Washington, DC: Task Force on Black and Minority Health, Department of Health and Human Services.

Hill, L., A. Rao, S. Artiga, and U. Ranji. 2024. *Racial disparities in maternal and infant health: Current status and efforts to address them.* KFF, October 25. https://www.kff.org/racial-equity-and-health-policy/issue-brief/racial-disparities-in-maternal-and-infant-health-current-status-and-efforts-to-address-them/ (accessed February 19, 2025).

Honeycutt, A. A., T. Hoerger, A. Hardee, L. Brown, K. Smith, and RTI International. 2011. *An assessment of the state of the art for measuring burden of illness.* Report prepared for Ansalan Stewart, U.S. Department of Health and Human Services. https://aspe.hhs.gov/sites/default/files/private/pdf/76381/index.pdf (accessed April 11, 2025).

Hoos, A., J. Anderson, M. Boutin, L. Dewulf, J. Geissler, G. Johnston, A. Joos, M. Metcalf, J. Regnante, I. Sargeant, R. F. Schneider, V. Todaro, and G. Tougas. 2015. Partnering with patients in the development and lifecycle of medicines: A call for action. *Therapeutic Innovation & Regulatory Science* 49(6):929–939.

Hyder, A. A., G. Rotllant, and R. H. Morrow. 1998. Measuring the burden of disease: Healthy life-years. *American Journal of Public Health* 88(2):196–202.

ICER (Institute for Clinical and Economic Review). 2020. *2020-2023 value assessment framework.* Boston, MA: ICER.

IHME (Institute for Health Metrics and Evaluation). n.d. *GBD history.* https://www.healthdata.org/research-analysis/about-gbd/history (accessed May 15, 2025).

IOM (Institute of Medicine). 1988. *Homelessness, health, and human needs.* Washington, DC: National Academy Press.

IOM. 1998a. *Scientific opportunities and public needs: Improving priority setting and public input at the National Institutes of Health.* Washington, DC: National Academy Press.

IOM. 1998b. *Summarizing population health: Directions for the development and application of population metrics.* Washington, DC: National Academy Press.

IOM. 2003. *Unequal treatment: Confronting racial and ethnic disparities in health care.* Washington, DC: The National Academies Press.

Jung, Y. L., J. Hwang, and H. S. Yoo. 2020. Disease burden metrics and the innovations of leading pharmaceutical companies: A global and regional comparative study. *Globalization and Health* 16(1):80.

Kanade, R. V., R. W. M. Van Deursen, K. Harding, and P. Price. 2006. Walking performance in people with diabetic neuropathy: Benefits and threats. *Diabetologia* 49(8):1747–1754.

Kaplan, R. M., and R. D. Hays. 2022. Health-related quality of life measurement in public health. *Annual Review of Public Health* 43:355–373.

Kaze, A. D., B. G. Jaar, G. C. Fonarow, and J. B. Echouffo-Tcheugui. 2022. Diabetic kidney disease and risk of incident stroke among adults with type 2 diabetes. *BMC Medicine* 20(1):127.

Kerr, G. H., A. van Donkelaar, R. V. Martin, M. Brauer, K. Bukart, S. Wozniak, D. L. Goldberg, and S. C. Anenberg. 2024. Increasing racial and ethnic disparities in ambient air pollution-attributable morbidity and mortality in the United States. *Environmental Health Perspectives* 132(3):037002.

Khaledi, M., F. Haghighatdoost, A. Feizi, and A. Aminorroaya. 2019. The prevalence of comorbid depression in patients with type 2 diabetes: An updated systematic review and meta-analysis on huge number of observational studies. *Acta Diabetologica* 56(6):631–650.

Khullar, D., and D. A. Chokshi. 2018. Health, income, & poverty: Where we are & what could help. *Health Affairs*, October 4. https://www.healthaffairs.org/content/briefs/health-income-poverty-we-could-help (accessed April 18, 2025).

Kiptinness, C., A. P. Kuo, A. M. Reedy, C. C. Johnson, K. Ngure, A. D. Wagner, and K. F. Ortblad. 2022. Examining the use of HIV self-testing to support prep delivery: A systematic literature review. *Current HIV/AIDS Reports* 19(5):394–408.

Klein, R. 1995. Hyperglycemie and microvascular and macrovascular disease in diabetes. *Diabetes Care* 18(2):258–268.

Krebber, A. M., L. M. Buffart, G. Kleijn, I. C. Riepma, R. de Bree, C. R. Leemans, A. Becker, J. Brug, A. van Straten, P. Cuijpers, and I. M. Verdonck-de Leeuw. 2014. Prevalence of depression in cancer patients: A meta-analysis of diagnostic interviews and self-report instruments. *Psychooncology* 23(2):121–130.

Lakatos, P. L., and L. Lakatos. 2008. Risk for colorectal cancer in ulcerative colitis: Changes, causes and management strategies. *World Journal of Gastroenterology* 14(25):3937–3947.

Lanar, S., C. Acquadro, J. Seaton, I. Savre, and B. Arnould. 2020. To what degree are orphan drugs patient-centered? A review of the current state of clinical research in rare diseases. *Orphanet Journal of Rare Diseases* 15(1):134.

Landovitz, R. J., D. Donnell, M. E. Clement, B. Hanscom, L. Cottle, L. Coelho, R. Cabello, S. Chariyalertsak, E. F. Dunne, I. Frank, J. A. Gallardo-Cartagena, A. H. Gaur, P. Gonzales, H. V. Tran, J. C. Hinojosa, E. G. Kallas, C. F. Kelley, M. H. Losso, J. V. Madruga, K. Middelkoop, N. Phanuphak, B. Santos, O. Sued, J. V. Huamaní, E. T. Overton, S. Swaminathan, C. d. Rio, R. M. Gulick, P. Richardson, P. Sullivan, E. Piwowar-Manning, M. Marzinke, C. Hendrix, M. Li, Z. Wang, J. Marrazzo, E. Daar, A. Asmelash, T. T. Brown, P. Anderson, S. H. Eshleman, M. Bryan, C. Blanchette, J. Lucas, C. Psaros, S. Safren, J. Sugarman, H. Scott, J. J. Eron, S. D. Fields, N. D. Sista, K. Gomez-Feliciano, A. Jennings, R. M. Kofron, T. H. Holtz, K. Shin, J. F. Rooney, K. Y. Smith, W. Spreen, D. Margolis, A. Rinehart, A. Adeyeye, M. S. Cohen, M. McCauley, and B. Grinsztejn. 2021. Cabotegravir for HIV prevention in cisgender men and transgender women. *New England Journal of Medicine* 385(7):595–608

Lapin, B. R. 2020. Considerations for reporting and reviewing studies including health-related quality of life. *Chest* 158(1):S49–S56.

Leininger, L. J., M. Tomaino, and E. Meara. 2023. Health-related quality of life in high-cost, high-need populations. *American Journal of Managed Care* 29(7):362–368.

Lodato, E., and W. Kaplan. 2013. *Priority medicines for Europe and the world: 2013 update report.* Geneva, Switzerland: World Health Organization. Pp. 68–74.

Lu, M. C., H. R. Guo, M. C. Lin, H. Livneh, N. S. Lai, and T. Y. Tsai. 2016. Bidirectional associations between rheumatoid arthritis and depression: A nationwide longitudinal study. *Science Reports* 6:20647.

M-CERSI (University of Maryland Center of Excellence in Regulatory Science and Innovation). 2025. *Home page.* https://cersi.umd.edu/ (accessed March 10, 2025).

Mitchell, A. J., B. Sheth, J. Gill, M. Yadegarfar, B. Stubbs, M. Yadegarfar, and N. Meader. 2017. Prevalence and predictors of post-stroke mood disorders: A meta-analysis and meta-regression of depression, anxiety and adjustment disorder. *General Hospital Psychiatry* 47:48–60.

Momen, N. C., O. Plana-Ripoll, E. Agerbo, M. E. Benros, A. D. Børglum, M. K. Christensen, S. Dalsgaard, L. Degenhardt, P. de Jonge, J. P. G. Debost, M. Fenger-Grøn, J. M. Gunn, K. M. Iburg, L. V. Kessing, R. C. Kessler, T. M. Laursen, C. C. W. Lim, O. Mors, P. B. Mortensen, K. L. Musliner, M. Nordentoft, C. B. Pedersen, L. V. Petersen, A. R. Ribe, A. M. Roest, S. Saha, A. J. Schork, K. M. Scott, C. Sievert, H. J. Sørensen, T. J. Stedman, M. Vestergaard, B. Vilhjalmsson, T. Werge, N. Weye, H. A. Whiteford, A. Prior, and J. J. McGrath. 2020. Association between mental disorders and subsequent medical conditions. *New England Journal of Medicine* 382(18):1721–1731.

Morgan, A. L., F. A. Masoudi, E. P. Havranek, P. G. Jones, P. N. Peterson, H. M. Krumholz, J. A. Spertus, and J. S. Rumsfeld. 2006. Difficulty taking medications, depression, and health status in heart failure patients. *Journal of Cardiac Failure* 12(1):54–60.

Mossadeghi, B., R. Caixeta, D. Ondarsuhu, S. Luciani, I. R. Hambleton, and A. J. M. Hennis. 2023. Multimorbidity and social determinants of health in the U.S. prior to the COVID-19 pandemic and implications for health outcomes: A cross-sectional analysis based on NHANES 2017–2018. *BMC Public Health* 23(1):887.

Murray, C. J. L., J. A. Salomon, C. D. Mathers, A. D. Lopez, and World Health Organization. 2002. *Summary measures of population health: Concepts, ethics, measurement and applications.* Geneva, Switzerland: World Health Organization.

Murray, C. J. L. 2022. The global burden of disease study at 30 years. *Nature Medicine* 28(10):2019–2026.

NASEM (National Academies of Sciences, Engineering, and Medicine). 2024. *Ending unequal treatment: Strategies to achieve equitable health care and optimal health for all.* Washington, DC: The National Academies Press.

Nayak, R. K., J. Avorn, and A. S. Kesselheim. 2019. Public sector financial support for late stage discovery of new drugs in the United States: Cohort study. *BMJ* 367:l5766.

Neumann, P. J., and J. T. Cohen. 2018. QALYs in 2018—Advantages and concerns. *JAMA* 319(24):2473–2474.

NIDDK (National Institute of Diabetes and Digestive and Kidney Diseases). 2024. *Diabetes statistics.* https://www.niddk.nih.gov/health-information/health-statistics/diabetes-statistics (accessed October 30, 2024).

Nuako, A., J. Liu, G. Pham, N. Smock, A. James, T. Baker, L. Bierut, G. Colditz, and L.-S. Chen. 2022. Quantifying rural disparity in healthcare utilization in the United States: Analysis of a large midwestern healthcare system. *PLoS ONE* 17(2):e0263718.

Ó Murchu, É., L. Marshall, C. Teljeur, P. Harrington, C. Hayes, P. Moran, and M. Ryan. 2022. Oral pre-exposure prophylaxis (PrEP) to prevent HIV: A systematic review and meta-analysis of clinical effectiveness, safety, adherence and risk compensation in all populations. *BMJ Open* 12(5):e048478.

O'Day, K., D. J. Mezzio, and P. H. Xcenda. 2021. Demystifying ICER's equal value of life years gained metric. *Value & Outcomes Spotlight* 7(1):26–28.

OECD (Organisation for Economic Co-operation and Development). 2022. *Avoidable mortality: OECD/Eurostat lists of preventable and treatable causes of death*. Paris, France: Organisation for Economic Co-operation and Development. https://www.oecd.org/content/dam/oecd/en/data/datasets/oecd-health-statistics/avoidable-mortality-2019-joint-oecd-eurostat-list-preventable-treatable-causes-of-death.pdf (accessed May 29, 2025).

Olfson, M., S. C. Marcus, J. Wilk, and J. C. West. 2006. Awareness of illness and nonadherence to antipsychotic medications among persons with schizophrenia. *Psychiatric Services* 57(2):205–211.

Ormel, J., S. D. Hollon, R. C. Kessler, P. Cuijpers, and S. M. Monroe. 2022. More treatment but no less depression: The treatment-prevalence paradox. *Clinical Psychology Review* 91:102111.

Ouellette, L. L., and B. N. Sampat. 2024. Using Bayh-Dole Act march-in rights to lower U.S. drug prices. *JAMA Health Forum* 5(11):e243775.

Pan, A., Q. Sun, O. I. Okereke, K. M. Rexrode, and F. B. Hu. 2011. Depression and risk of stroke morbidity and mortality. JAMA 306(11):1241.

Parker, E. D., J. Lin, T. Mahoney, N. Ume, G. Yang, R. A. Gabbay, N. A. Elsayed, and R. R. Bannuru. 2024. Economic costs of diabetes in the U.S. in 2022. *Diabetes Care* 47(1):26–43.

Pascoe, J. M., D. L. Wood, J. H. Duffee, A. Kuo, M. Yogman, N. Bauer, T. B. Gambon, A. Lavin, K. M. Lemmon, G. Mattson, J. R. Rafferty, L. S. Wissow, B. A. Gitterman, P. J. Flanagan, W. H. Cotton, K. J. Dilley, A. E. Green, V. A. Keane, S. D. Krugman, J. M. Linton, C. D. McKelvey, and J. L. Nelson. 2016. Mediators and adverse effects of child poverty in the United States. *Pediatrics* 137(4):e20160340.

Patients as Partners. 2023. *Novartis' bold vision to change how the entire sector engages patients*. https://theconferenceforum.org/editorial/novartis-global-head-of-patient-engagements-bold-vision-to-change-how-the-entire-sector-engages-patients/ (accessed April 12, 2025).

PCORI (Patient-Centered Outcomes Research Institute). n.d. *Explore our portfolio*. https://www.pcori.org/explore-our-portfolio (accessed March 19, 2025).

Powder, J. 2022. *A prescription for PrEP uptake*. https://publichealth.jhu.edu/2022/a-prescription-for-prep-uptake (accessed May 30, 2025).

Rand, L. Z., and A. S. Kesselheim. 2021. Controversy over using quality adjusted life years in cost-effectiveness analyses: A systematic literature review. *Health Affairs (Millwood)* 40(9):1402–1410.

Rapsey, C. M., C. C. W. Lim, A. Al-Hamzawi, J. Alonso, R. Bruffaerts, J. M. Caldas-De-Almeida, S. Florescu, G. De Girolamo, C. Hu, R. C. Kessler, V. Kovess-Masfety, D. Levinson, M. E. Medina-Mora, S. Murphy, Y. Ono, M. Piazza, J. Posada-Villa, M. Ten Have, B. Wojtyniak, and K. M. Scott. 2015. Associations between DSM-IV mental disorders and subsequent COPD diagnosis. *Journal of Psychosomatic Research* 79(5):333–339.

Rees, C. A., M. C. Monuteaux, V. Herdell, E. W. Fleegler, and F. T. Bourgeois. 2021. Correlation between National Institutes of Health funding for pediatric research and pediatric disease burden in the U.S. *JAMA Pediatrics* 175(12):1236–1243.

Research!America. 2022. *U.S. investments in medical and health research and development: 2016-2020*. https://www.researchamerica.org/wp-content/uploads/2022/09/ResearchAmerica-Investment-Report.Final_.January-2022-1.pdf (accessed April 12, 2025).

Salomon, J. A., T. Vos, D. R. Hogan, M. Gagnon, M. Naghavi, A. Mokdad, N. Begum, R. Shah, M. Karyana, S. Kosen, M. R. Farje, G. Moncada, A. Dutta, S. Sazawal, A. Dyer, J. Seiler, V. Aboyans, L. Baker, A. Baxter, E. J. Benjamin, K. Bhalla, A. B. Abdulhak, F. Blyth, R. Bourne, T. Braithwaite, P. Brooks, T. S. Brugha, C. Bryan-Hancock, R. Buchbinder, P. Burney, B. Calabria, H. Chen, S. S. Chugh, R. Cooley, M. H. Criqui, M. Cross, K. C. Dabhadkar, N. Dahodwala, A. Davis, L. Degenhardt, C. Díaz-Torné, E. R. Dorsey, T. Driscoll, K. Edmond, A. Elbaz, M. Ezzati, V. Feigin, C. P. Ferri, A. D. Flaxman, L. Flood, M. Fransen, K. Fuse, B. J. Gabbe, R. F. Gillum, J. Haagsma, J. E. Harrison, R. Havmoeller, R. J. Hay, A. Hel-Baqui, H. W. Hoek, H. Hoffman, E. Hogeland, D. Hoy, D. Jarvis, J. B. Jonas, G. Karthikeyan, L. M. Knowlton, T. Lathlean, J. L. Leasher, S. S. Lim, S. E. Lipshultz, A. D. Lopez, R. Lozano, R. Lyons, R. Malekzadeh, W. Marcenes, L. March, D. J. Margolis, N. McGill, J. McGrath, G. A. Mensah, A.-C. Meyer, C. Michaud, A. Moran, R. Mori, M. E. Murdoch, L. Naldi, C. R. Newton, R. Norman, S. B. Omer, R. Osborne, N. Pearce, F. Perez-Ruiz, N. Perico, K. Pesudovs, D. Phillips, F. Pourmalek, M. Prince, J. T. Rehm, G. Remuzzi, K. Richardson, R. Room, S. Saha, U. Sampson, L. Sanchez-Riera, M. Segui-Gomez, S. Shahraz, K. Shibuya, D. Singh, K. Sliwa, E. Smith, I. Soerjomataram, T. Steiner, W. A. Stolk, L. J. Stovner, C. Sudfeld, H. R. Taylor, I. M. Tleyjeh, M. J. Van Der Werf, W. L. Watson, D. J. Weatherall, R. Weintraub, M. G. Weisskopf, H. Whiteford, J. D. Wilkinson, A. D. Woolf, Z.-J. Zheng, and C. J. Murray. 2012. Common values in assessing health outcomes from disease and injury: Disability weights measurement study for the Global Burden of Disease Study 2010. *Lancet* 380(9859):2129–2143.

Sarnak, M. J., K. Amann, S. Bangalore, J. L. Cavalcante, D. M. Charytan, J. C. Craig, J. S. Gill, M. A. Hlatky, A. G. Jardine, U. Landmesser, L. K. Newby, C. A. Herzog, M. Cheung, D. C. Wheeler, W. C. Winkelmayer, T. H. Marwick, D. Banerjee, C. Briguori, T. I. Chang, C.-L. Chen, C. R. deFilippi, X. Ding, C. J. Ferro, J. Gill, M. Gössl, N. M. Isbel, H. Ishii, M. J. Jardine, P. A. Kalra, G. Laufer, K. L. Lentine, K. Lobdell, C. E. Lok, G. M. London, J. Małyszko, P. B. Mark, M. Marwan, Y. Nie, P. S. Parfrey, R. Pecoits-Filho, H. Pilmore, W. Y. Qunibi, P. Raggi, M. Rattazzi, P. Rossignol, J. Ruturi, C. Sabanayagam, C. M. Shanahan, G. R. Shroff, R. Shroff, A. C. Webster, D. E. Weiner, S. Winther, A. C. Wiseman, A. Yip, and A. Zarbock. 2019. Chronic kidney disease and coronary artery disease: JACC state-of-the-art review. *Journal of the American College of Cardiology* 74(14):1823–1838.

Schuch, F., D. Vancampfort, J. Firth, S. Rosenbaum, P. Ward, T. Reichert, N. C. Bagatini, R. Bgeginski, and B. Stubbs. 2017. Physical activity and sedentary behavior in people with major depressive disorder: A systematic review and meta-analysis. *Journal of Affective Disorders* 210:139–150.

Scott, K. M., C. Lim, A. Al-Hamzawi, J. Alonso, R. Bruffaerts, J. M. Caldas-de-Almeida, S. Florescu, G. de Girolamo, C. Hu, P. de Jonge, N. Kawakami, M. E. Medina-Mora, J. Moskalewicz, F. Navarro-Mateu, S. O'Neill, M. Piazza, J. Posada-Villa, Y. Torres, and R. C. Kessler. 2016. Association of mental disorders with subsequent chronic physical conditions: World mental health surveys from 17 countries. *JAMA Psychiatry* 73(2):150–158.

Shrivastav, M. T., Z. Malik, and Somlata. 2021. Revisiting drug development against the neglected tropical disease, amebiasis. *Frontiers in Cellular and Infection Microbiology* 10:628257.

Simoens, S., and I. Huys. 2022. How much do the public sector and the private sector contribute to biopharmaceutical R&D? *Drug Discovery Today* 27(4):939–945.

SiRM (Strategies in Regulated Markets), L.E.K. Consulting, and RAND Europe. 2022. *The financial ecosystem of pharmaceutical R&D: An evidence base to inform further dialogue.* https://www.rand.org/content/dam/rand/pubs/external_publications/EP60000/EP68954/RAND_EP68954.pdf (accessed May 29, 2025).

Slabaugh, S. L., M. Shah, M. Zack, L. Happe, T. Cordier, E. Havens, E. Davidson, M. Miao, T. Prewitt, and H. Jia. 2017. Leveraging health-related quality of life in population health management: The case for healthy days. *Population Health Management* 20(1):13–22.

Spencer, A., O. Rivero-Arias, R. Wong, A. Tsuchiya, H. Bleichrodt, R. T. Edwards, R. Norman, A. Lloyd, and P. Clarke. 2022. The QALY at 50: One story many voices. *Social Science & Medicine* 296:114653.

Stevens, A. J., J. J. Jensen, K. Wyller, P. C. Kilgore, S. Chatterjee, and M. L. Rohrbaugh. 2011. The role of public-sector research in the discovery of drugs and vaccines. *New England Journal of Medicine* 364(6):535–541.

Stockmann, C., A. L. Hersh, C. M. Sherwin, and M. G. Spigarelli. 2014. Alignment of United States funding for cardiovascular disease research with deaths, years of life lost, and hospitalizations. *International Journal of Cardiology* 172(1):e19–e21.

Tonin, F. S., I. Aznar-Lou, V. M. Pontinha, R. Pontarolo, and F. Fernandez-Llimos. 2021. Principles of pharmacoeconomic analysis: The case of pharmacist-led interventions. *Pharmacy Practice* 19(1):2302.

Touré, M., C. R. C. Kouakou, and T. G. Poder. 2021. Dimensions used in instruments for QALY calculation: A systematic review. *International Journal of Environmental Research and Public Health* 18(9):4428.

Visaria, J., N. N. Iyer, A. D. Raval, S. X. Kong, T. Hobbs, J. Bouchard, D. M. Kern, and V. J. Willey. 2020. Healthcare costs of diabetes and microvascular and macrovascular disease in individuals with incident type 2 diabetes mellitus: A ten-year longitudinal study. *ClinicoEconomics and Outcomes Research* 12:423–434.

Vreman, R., I. Heikkinen, A. Schuurman, C. Sapede, J. Llinares, N. Hedberg, D. Athanasiou, J. Grueger, H. Leufkens, and W. Goettsch. 2019. Unmet medical need: An introduction to definitions and stakeholder perceptions. *Value in Health* 22.

Waldron, J. 2024. Puretech's lung fibrosis drug slows decline in phase 2 trial. *Fierce Biotech*. https://www.fiercebiotech.com/biotech/puretechs-lung-fibrosis-drug-slows-decline-phase-2-trial (accessed May 20, 2025).

Walker, J., K. Burke, M. Wanat, R. Fisher, J. Fielding, A. Mulick, S. Puntis, J. Sharpe, M. D. Esposti, E. Harriss, C. Frost, and M. Sharpe. 2018. The prevalence of depression in general hospital inpatients: A systematic review and meta-analysis of interview-based studies. *Psychological Medicine* 48(14):2285–2298.

Wang, J., X. Wu, W. Lai, E. Long, X. Zhang, W. Li, Y. Zhu, C. Chen, X. Zhong, Z. Liu, D. Wang, and H. Lin. 2017. Prevalence of depression and depressive symptoms among outpatients: A systematic review and meta-analysis. *BMJ Open* 7(8):e017173.

WHO (World Health Organization). 2016. *WHO manual for estimating the economic burden of seasonal influenza.* Geneva, Switzerland: World Health Organization. http://www.who.int/immunization/research/development/influenza_maternal_immunization/en/index2.html (accessed January 23, 2025).

WHO. 2021. *New cost-effectiveness updates from WHO-CHOICE.* https://www.who.int/news-room/feature-stories/detail/new-cost-effectiveness-updates-from-who-choice (accessed March 21, 2025).

World Bank. 1993. *World development report 1993: Investing in health.* Washington, DC: World Bank.

Yu, M., X. Zhang, F. Lu, and L. Fang. 2015. Depression and risk for diabetes: A meta-analysis. *Canadian Journal of Diabetes* 39(4):266–272.

Zack, M. M. 2013. Health-related quality of life - United States, 2006 and 2010. *Morbidity and Mortality Weekly Report* 62(3):105–111.

3

Degree and Patterns of Mismatch Between U.S. Disease Burden and Public and Private Investment in Innovative Therapeutic Development

Building on Chapter 2, which defined key constructs needed to assess mismatches between disease burden and investment in innovation, this chapter seeks to review the existing empirical data that were accessible to the committee and answer the question of what is currently known about the patterns of mismatch between U.S. disease burden and investment. Several groups have attempted to study the mismatch between disease burden and investment in therapeutic development and to develop a list of areas where future investments are needed, and the following sections provide an overview of some of those efforts. However, it should be noted that such lists of underinvested disease areas vary depending on the specific data, methodology, and values used to develop them. Many existing lists prioritize one set of criteria or do not account for some, often hard-to-measure, factors. For example, as discussed in Chapter 2, disease burden is often estimated via total disability-adjusted life-years (DALYs); however, disease burden has multiple dimensions. Data aggregation poses another challenge—that is, existing data on disease burden may use categories for disease causes that do not match classifications for therapeutic areas, which complicates the assessment of alignment. One aspect of this challenge is that the burden of disease is often assessed for broad categories that encompass many diseases and lack the granularity necessary to identify mismatch for more specific conditions or to understand the nuances that contributed to a mismatch.

Recognizing the limitations of existing data, the committee began by reviewing findings from the most commonly used paradigm for assessment investment mismatch, which compares total burden of disease to public research investment, focusing on the National Institutes of Health (NIH) as the primary funder of biomedical research in the United States. The chapter proceeds with a discussion of private investment and closes with commentary on additional nuances to take into account when assessing mismatch between disease burden and investment. Throughout, the committee highlights limitations of the data available for this exercise.

PUBLIC INVESTMENT IN THERAPEUTIC DEVELOPMENT

As described in Chapter 2, the public sector, through federal agencies such as NIH, has contributed significantly to drug development, particularly through a focus on basic science and discovery research (see Chapter 2, section "Investment in Therapeutic Innovation"). Driving the agency's research agenda, NIH's mission is to "seek fundamental knowledge about the nature and behavior of living systems and the application of that knowledge to enhance health, lengthen life, and reduce illness and disability" (NIH, 2024). The agency is focused on supporting innovation, creativity, and science in advancing fundamental knowledge on human health. Its work supports a spectrum of research on the causes, diagnosis, prevention, and cure of human diseases. NIH activities cover a wide range of basic, clinical, and translational research, focused on particular diseases, areas of human health and development, or more fundamental aspects of biology and behavior (Congressional Research Service, 2023).

NIH considers disease burden rates when determining funding priorities, specifically, using the Research, Condition, and Disease Categorization (RCDC) system, which publicly reports funding for medical research across diseases and conditions (NIH RePORT, n.d.). NIH's funding decisions, including about biopharmaceutical research, are made through a dual-level peer-review process that prioritizes support of scientific ideas with "the greatest potential impact to improve human health or otherwise advance biomedical research" (NIH, 2023).

In fiscal year (FY) 2024, NIH received program-level funding totaling over $47.311 billion, a decrease in its overall program level in nominal dollars for the first time since FY2013 (Congressional Research Service, 2024). The FY2025 budget maintains NIH and Advanced Research Projects Agency for Health (ARPA-H) program funding at approximately the same level as FY2024.[1] However, the President's proposed budget for FY2026 calls for a nearly $18 billion reduction to NIH, which would amount to a roughly 40 percent cut (OMB, 2025).

---

[1] Full-Year Continuing Appropriations and Extensions Act, 2025. Public Law 119-4, 119th Congress (March 15, 2025).

Several groups have analyzed NIH funding information to assess how well the allocations align with disease burden (e.g., Ballreich et al., 2021; Gillum et al., 2011; Rees et al., 2021). The dominant paradigm in these assessments is to compare total DALYs versus NIH funding to identify diseases that have disproportionately low investment. In one example published in 2021, an analysis of NIH funding by disease category examined DALYs in 2008 and 2019 to determine alignment with funding for 46 diseases (Ballreich et al., 2021). These 46 diseases represented more than 66 percent of all DALYs in both 2008 and 2019, leaving out 34 percent of diseases that affect the U.S. population. The analysis found that NIH funding allocations appeared to shift minimally over 10 years, despite substantial changes in the contributions of different diseases to the overall burden of disease. The authors recommended, "NIH should examine the allocation process to ensure NIH investments are responsive to changes in the health of the population" (Ballreich et al., 2021).

The authors identified three diseases with substantially lower funding (eating disorders, uterine cancer, and psoriasis) relative to burden across both 2008 and 2019, and three diseases with higher funding (HIV/AIDS, digestive diseases, and urologic diseases). Their analysis of the change in funding from 2008 to 2019 showed that funding for Alzheimer's and dementia increased the most (> 350 percent increase) and that funding for interpersonal violence, multiple sclerosis, Hodgkin lymphoma, and otitis media had the largest decreases (≥ 40 percent decrease); these changes were not proportional to the percent change in total DALYs, though they may reflect scientific and therapeutic developments in these areas during this period (Ballreich et al., 2021).

The committee analyzed publicly available data on disease burden and NIH funding in the years 2019–2021 to further inform its assessment of mismatch (Figure 3-1). Data on disease burden as measured by DALYs were collected from the Global Burden of Disease Dataset available through the Institute of Health Metrics and Evaluation (IHME). NIH funding information was gathered from the NIH RePORTER database. A ratio between NIH funding and the DALYs rate (DALYs per 100,000 population) was calculated to determine whether disease areas had a high, low, or proportional share of funding.[2]

This analysis identified the following diseases and conditions that had disproportionately low NIH funding relative to disease burden (DALY rate) in 2021: ischemic heart disease, low back pain, chronic obstructive pulmonary disease (COPD), headache disorders, neck pain, gallbladder and biliary diseases, and psoriasis. Some diseases had a higher share of funding than their disease burden would indicate, including Alzheimer's disease and other

---

[2] DALYs rate and NIH funding information were available for 59 disease areas for 2021, the most recent year for which both burden and funding information were known.

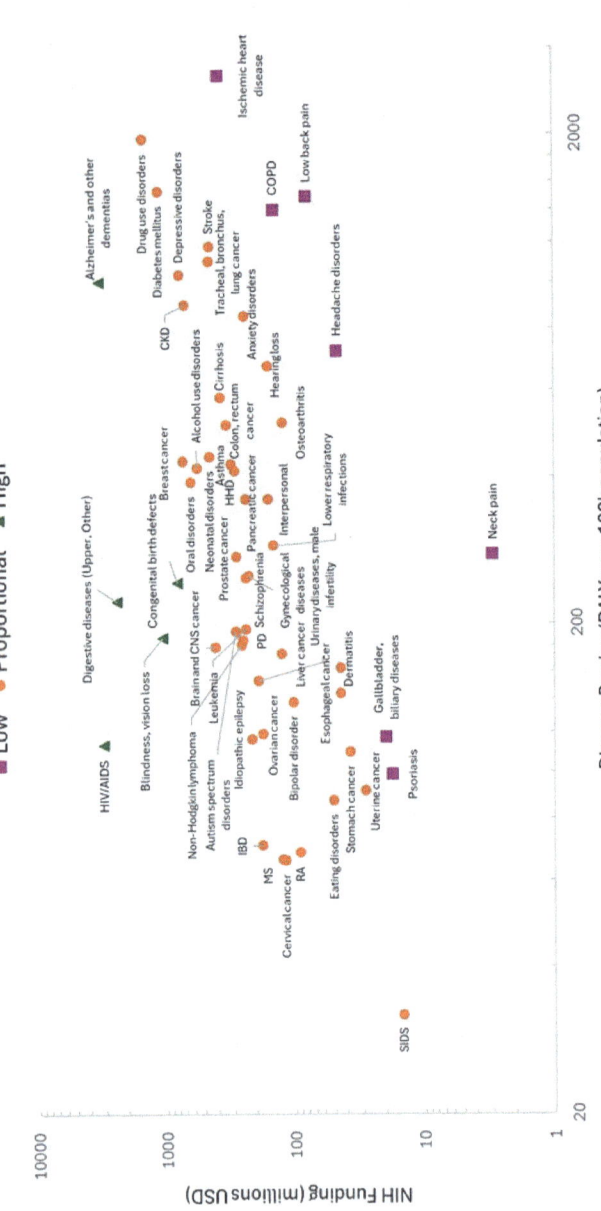

FIGURE 3-1 Comparison of NIH funding *vs.* disease burden in 2021.
NOTES: Purple squares indicate diseases with low funding to burden ratio. Green triangles indicate diseases with a high funding to burden ratio. Orange circles indicate relatively proportional funding to disease burden. CKD = chronic kidney disease; CNS = central nervous system; COPD = chronic obstructive pulmonary disease; HHD = hypertensive heart disease; IBD = inflammatory bowel disease; MS = multiple sclerosis; PD = Parkinson's disease; RA = rheumatoid arthritis; SIDS = sudden infant death syndrome. Not all diseases are represented in the plot.
SOURCE: Created using data from NIH and IHME data, 2021.

dementias, congenital birth defects, blindness and vision loss, digestive system diseases, and HIV/AIDS. Of note, these findings are relative to disease burden in the United States; however, funding may not be overweighted considering the global burden of HIV/AIDS, for example. Emphasizing the need for disaggregated data, the ratio of NIH funding relative to disease burden differs for different types of cancer. For example, brain and central nervous system cancers have higher investment than liver or esophageal cancers, despite comparable rates of disease burden. This may reflect differential unmet need profiles across these types of cancer, although it is difficult to say conclusively without additional data. It is also notable that neck pain, low back pain, and headache disorders appear to have lower public investment. This may be, in part, because pain is subjective and often idiopathic, making it challenging to study. Moreover, a condition like food allergies, which has been reported to affect more than 26 million people in the United States, was not included on this list of diseases (Gupta et al., 2019; Sansweet et al., 2024).

This evidence, together with prior analyses, indicates some misalignment between NIH funding and disease burden. COPD stands out as a condition that has relatively low public investment across many of these studies; whereas, HIV/AIDS and Alzheimer's disease and other neurological diseases, while having a large disease burden, have appeared in multiple instances to have relatively high investment compared with burden. Misalignment may be a result, in part, of congressional appropriations made for certain conditions, such as Alzheimer's disease and dementia, and advocacy for specific diseases could play a role in their relative funding level (Ballreich et al., 2021; Best, 2012). (See Chapter 5, section "NIH Funding Process" for more information about how NIH funding is allocated.)

Compounding this misalignment is the fact that funding for research on diseases of significant public interest may be neglected by private funding owing to its potential for small market share. For example, rare diseases affect a small population with potential smaller market share and thus may not be a focus of private research and development (R&D) absent market incentives, though there has been considerable progress in developing novel treatments for narrow indications in recent years with 26 of 50 novel drug approvals in 2024 being for rare diseases (FDA, 2025). Taken together, the committee found that disease burden and unmet medical need are multidimensional and challenging to measure, which suggests the need for multiple measures to effectively assess alignment or mismatch among these factors. A data repository that compiles multiple metrics of disease burden and unmet need would enable different organizations to access relevant data and create lists that reflect their priorities and values. For example, prioritizing reducing disparities across populations would require information on individual burden or data aggregated by relevant sociodemographic groups, not only population burden.

Limitations of Using NIH Funding Data to Assess Mismatch

There are several known limitations of this approach of comparing total DALYs to NIH funding to assess the mismatch between burden and investment. The data are imperfect—some disease areas may be missing or unavailable in different analyses, and it can be challenging to align disease burden measurements with NIH funding categories, which can lead to variation and uncertainty in these results. Additionally, some investments in basic science that benefit multiple disease categories are typically not captured separately for each disease, which adds the complexity to categorizing the investment allocation by disease. Moreover, this simple comparison of DALYs and NIH funding reduces complex, multidimensional concepts, such as burden (see Chapter 2), to a single dimension and metric. It captures only a snapshot of disease burden at one point in time. For some diseases like Alzheimer's disease, the projected disease burden is higher than current burden, potentially warranting higher investments in preclinical research now to help address projected unmet need for future populations.

On the investment side, a focus on NIH, while traditionally the largest public funder of biomedical research, excludes the contributions of other public funding sources, such as the U.S. Department of Defense and the Biomedical Advanced Research and Development Authority (BARDA), to biomedical R&D. In 2021, for example, BARDA had a budget of $1.4 billion to advance medical countermeasures for responding to health threats.[3] In addition, analyzing NIH funding relates to only part of the product development pipeline and omits information about private-sector investment. Analyzing DALYs versus NIH funding also does not account for unmet need and innovation, key components of this committee's statement of task. However, there are a number of obstacles to operationalizing a more nuanced, complex framework—not least of which is availability of the data required. In addition, priority setting becomes far more challenging with more dimensions and criteria. As a next step, the committee assessed the role of private-sector funding.

PRIVATE-SECTOR FUNDING AND PRIORITIES FOR BIOPHARMACEUTICAL RESEARCH

Data indicate that private funding for biopharmaceutical development has been increasing over time. For example, the share of U.S. medical research funded by industry grew from 46 percent in 1994 to 58 percent in 2012, with industry providing the primary funding for late-phase clinical

---

[3] https://aspr.hhs.gov/AboutASPR/BudgetandFunding/Pages/BudgetandFundingFY2021.aspx (accessed April 21, 2025).

trials (Moses et al., 2015). Another study found that from 2006 to 2014, the number of industry-funded clinical trials registered in ClinicalTrials.gov increased by 43 percent, while the number of NIH-funded trials decreased by 28 percent (Ehrhardt et al., 2015). Measuring the relative contributions of the private and public sector to drug development is challenging, but one study suggests that when accounting for basic research, NIH investment in drugs approved from 2010 to 2019 was not less than private-sector funding (Galkina Cleary et al., 2023). NIH funding is primarily used to support public goods such as understanding the biological mechanisms of disease (Galkina Cleary et al., 2018), and the NIH also funds a significant number of phase I and II clinical trials in areas such as gene therapy (Kassir et al., 2020). However, these contributions are generally unpatentable, and late-stage patentable contributions are largely privately funded. For example, of the 1,213 patented drugs that were on the market in 2023, only 45 (4 percent) had any federally funded patents, and only 16 (1 percent) had solely federally funded patents (Ouellette and Sampat, 2024).

According to a 2023 report, significant funding from the pharmaceutical sector is devoted to oncology and neurology research. These products constitute the highest share of the R&D pipeline (see Figure 3-2). Particularly, oncology remains the focus of the pipeline, accounting for 38 percent or 2,331 products and growing at 10.5 percent compound annual growth rate over the last 5 years (IQVIA, 2023).

Venture capital (VC) funding accounts for approximately 10 percent of investment in biopharmaceutical R&D globally and plays a key role in funding early-stage, innovative ventures (SiRM et al., 2022). A 2024 study by Kang et al. analyzed VC funding patterns in pharmaceutical R&D from 2014 to 2024 and similarly found that the investment was concentrated in oncology and neurology/psychiatry. Cancer alone accounted for nearly 30 percent of VC deals in 2023, and the authors suggest that "FDA [Food and Drug Administration] and payment incentives may influence VC investments" in these therapeutic areas (Kang et al., 2024). In addition, approximately 75 percent of VC investments were focused on small-molecule drugs as compared to biologics or gene therapies, with this pattern relatively stable over the period 2014–2024 (Kang et al., 2024), though trends may change depending on legislation and other policy parameters. These investments in cancer affect half of all men and one-third of all women in the United States expected to be diagnosed with cancer in their lifetimes (NCI, n.d.). Funding for cancer research also contributes to improvements in the biological understanding of malignancy achieved in the last few years (Wang et al., 2023).

Interestingly, the study found that VC investments were concentrated on early-stage, particularly phase I, clinical trials, with increasing investment in phase I trials over the period analyzed. Phase I trials accounted

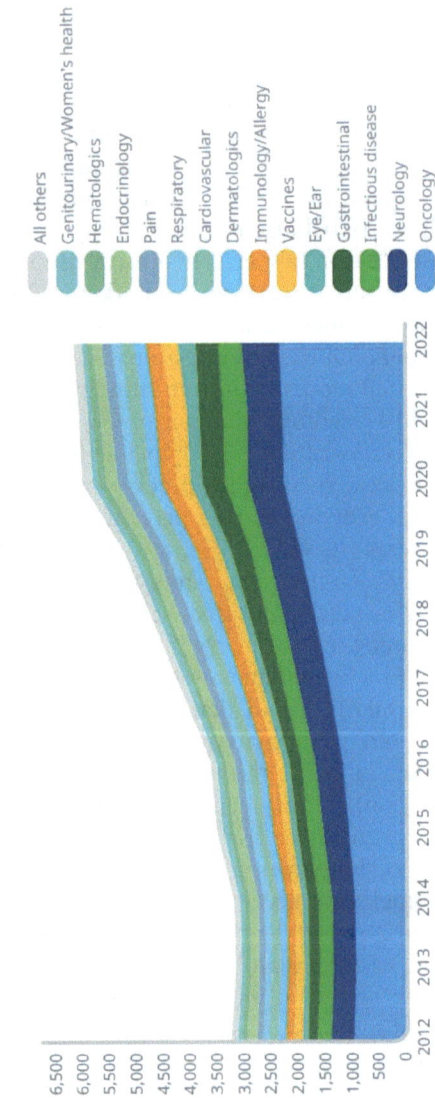

Growth in the clinical pipeline has remained flat since 2020, although 49% above 2017 levels

FIGURE 3-2 Number of pipeline products from phase I to regulatory submission by therapeutic drug class, 2012–2022.
NOTES: Includes drugs with an active research program, with phase determined by the highest phase of research regardless of indication. Oncology includes supportive care. Neurology includes central nervous system disorder treatments and mental health treatments but does not include pain management or anesthesia.
SOURCE: IQVIA, 2023.

for nearly half of VC deals by 2023 and 61.2 percent of deals in the first quarter of 2024 (Kang et al., 2024). Although phase I trials are risky and known to have the highest failure rates in drug development, the authors suggest that this trend may reflect strategic positioning (Kang et al., 2024). That is, as large pharmaceutical companies acquire biopharmaceutical companies at early stages, VC firms respond by investing earlier, despite the higher risk, to position such companies for acquisition and enhanced return on investment. Earlier exits may also be more profitable given the expense of and risk associated with later-stage clinical trials (Kang et al., 2024). Conducting a trial costs $25,000 or more per patient and phase 3 trials are the primary driver of R&D costs (Gandjour, 2024; Kantarjian et al., 2013; Light and Warburton, 2011). This can make raising capital for certain conditions, such as cardiovascular disease, difficult because there are already several generics on the market so prices must be low; however, expensive, long-term, large phase 3 trials are still required (Kocher and Roberts, 2014).

Furthermore, because VC firms want to invest in drugs that are likely to be acquired after phase 2 by larger pharmaceutical companies, they are more likely to invest in therapeutic areas that are a focus area of large pharmaceutical companies. Without the sales force, manufacturing, and customer service expertise already in place, it becomes more challenging to raise the additional funds required to build these critical functions. In the context of the committee's statement of task, these trends could exacerbate misalignment between investment in innovation and disease burden if early-stage R&D decisions are increasingly influenced by potential return on investment and market forces, rather than by public health needs.

Another recent IQVIA report provides additional insight into therapeutic innovation and new trends in pharmaceutical development since the Inflation Reduction Act (IRA) was passed in 2022, though these data and trends are still emerging. The report examined postapproval expansions, which typically extend drug indications to additional patient populations or conditions, from 2000 to 2023 and analyzed early data on the effects of the IRA's Medicare Drug Price Negotiation Program. The study found that postapproval expansions are widespread—approximately 50 percent of drugs received at least one postinitial approval expansion, and the pattern is relatively consistent across small molecules (52 percent) and biologics (47 percent) (IQVIA, 2025). Another study found that about 55 percent of cancer drugs receive approval for at least one supplemental indication (Stoelinga et al., 2024). Importantly, the innovation life cycle for a new drug is not complete at the time of initial approval (IQVIA, 2025).

With the IRA, which could change with new legislation, small molecules are subject to Medicare price negotiation after 9 years and biologics after 13 years, compressing the timeline to develop supplemental indications prior to possible price negotiation (see Chapter 5 for more detail).[4] Although it is possible that this change could disincentivize investment in indication expansions as IRA deadlines approach, most expansions occur within the first few years following initial approval (Stoelinga et al., 2024). Considering biologics for example, 33 percent of expansions happened after year 9 postapproval (IQVIA, 2025). Approximately 15 percent of expansions were secured after the IRA's price negotiation time frames of 9 or 13 years (IQVIA, 2025). Nonetheless, because clinical trials are lengthy and expensive, if new indications are identified closer to the negotiation deadline, sponsors may decide that investment is not worth it, especially in the context of some rare diseases, leaving potentially beneficial indications undeveloped. Given longstanding strategic considerations, the development of follow-on indications could change significantly depending on various policy parameters.

Importantly, negotiated prices consider R&D costs, as well as several other factors, and are not intended to eliminate profit; in fact, in the first round of negotiations, most of the negotiated Medicare prices remained substantially higher than prices abroad (Rome et al., 2024). Thus, developing supplemental indications should still offer strong returns for industry. However, to the extent that the IRA significantly affects decision making in the private sector about whether new indications are worth the investment in R&D, public funding may be necessary to support investigation of new off-label uses.

Distribution of Pharmaceutical Products Compared with Burden

In addition to the literature reviewed above, the committee also worked with Steve Lim, a professor of health metrics sciences and the senior director of science and engineering at IHME, who served as an unpaid consultant to the committee. The IHME research team shared in-progress data that were collected as part of its assessment of the alignment between disease burden and pharmaceutical development, using pharmaceutical products as a proxy for investment. The committee considered data from IHME comparing the distribution of pharmaceutical products in the development pipeline with the U.S. burden of disease (DALYs) projected in 2030 (Figures 3-3, 3-4). Briefly, data on drugs in the development pipeline were collected from a variety of databases (EvaluatePharma, Redbook, Micromedex, Martindale)

---

[4] An executive order from April 15, 2025, requested that the HHS secretary work with Congress to eliminate differences between the treatment of small molecules and biologics under the Medicare Drug Price Negotiation Program. https://www.whitehouse.gov/presidential-actions/2025/04/lowering-drug-prices-by-once-again-putting-americans-first/ (accessed May 22, 2025).

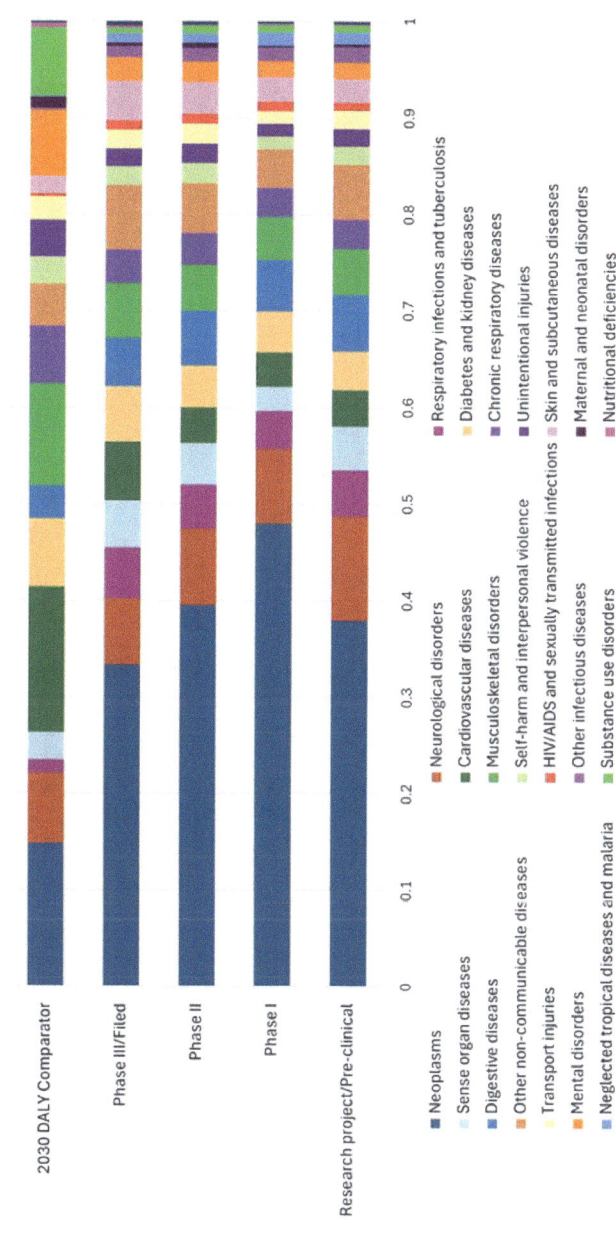

Causes Targeted by Products per Pipeline Phase

FIGURE 3-3 Pipeline products disaggregated by phase of product development.
NOTES: The top bar indicates the proportion of total U.S. DALYs that each of 22 disease categories contributes. The top bar provides a comparison to each of the other bars, which show the proportion of products in the development pipeline from preclinical research through phase III across all 6,576 pharmaceutical companies analyzed.
SOURCE: Adapted from IHME data, 2025.

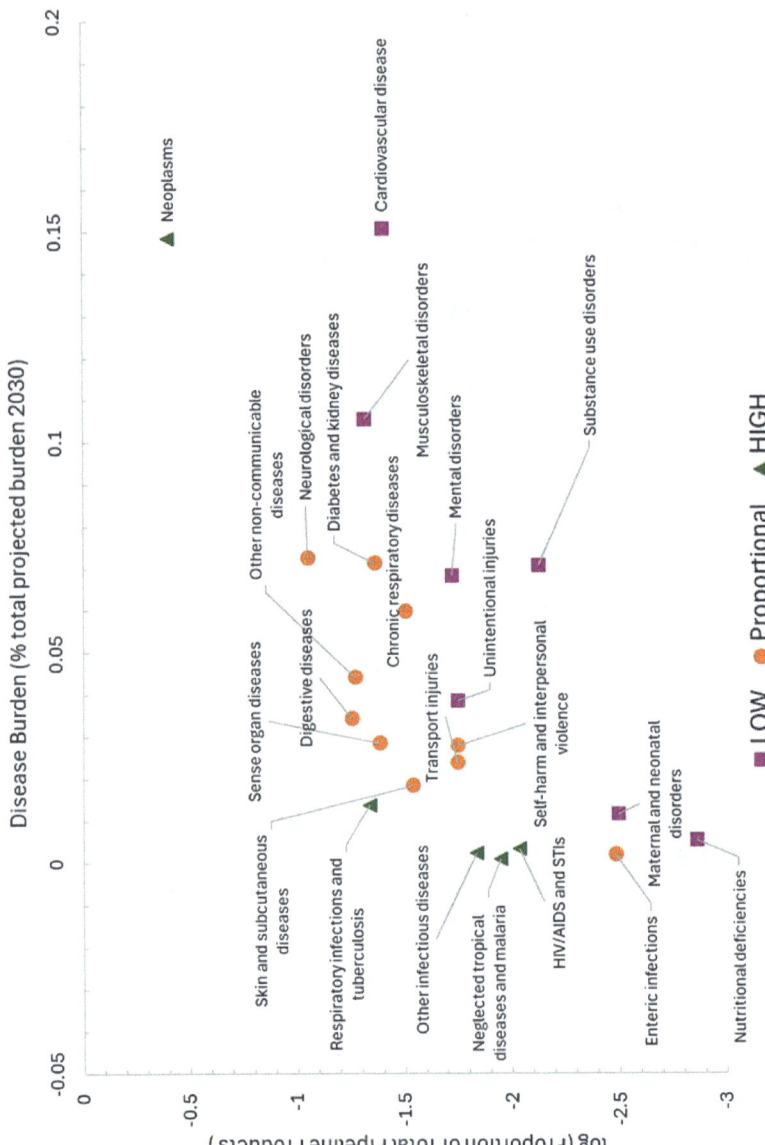

FIGURE 3-4 Total pipeline products *vs.* U.S. disease burden in 2030.
SOURCE: Adapted from IHME data, 2025.

for a total of 6,576 pharmaceutical companies.[5] ChatGPT was prompted to code, or match, prescribed drug use to most likely disease cause. The distribution of these drug–use pairs was compared to the distribution of DALYs across 22 disease areas to assess mismatch. (See Appendix D for more detailed methodology.)

The results indicate substantial private-sector investment in neoplasms, or tumors. This may be attributable in part to high unmet need in cancer treatment and the low rate of success in developing new effective treatments in oncology—potentially warranting greater investment. Policies, such as Medicare Part B reimbursement, also shape the incentive and decision-making structure around the development of oncology therapies. Neurological diseases also account for a large number of the treatments in development, though the investment appears relatively proportional to burden. Other areas with high investment relative to proportion of DALYs include HIV/AIDS and sexually transmitted infections, neglected tropical diseases, respiratory infections and tuberculosis, and other infectious diseases. For some of these diseases, such as HIV/AIDS, tropical diseases, and tuberculosis, investment could be responding to high *global* burden of disease.

Areas with comparatively low private investment are nutritional deficiencies, maternal and neonatal disorders, mental health disorders, substance use disorders, cardiovascular diseases, and unintentional injuries. Taking cardiovascular disease as an example, a number of factors could explain the seeming underinvestment. The clinical trials required are large, lengthy, and expensive, and generic treatments already on the market reduce market incentives for developing new therapies that further address residual unmet need. Although cardiovascular disease represents a large potential market for new treatments, the market is already partially satisfied by existing, effective treatments, and low-cost generics can limit uptake of newer, more expensive options. However, good therapeutic options may not be fully used, leaving a gap in unaddressed disease burden. While innovative therapies could be helpful, innovation may not be the primary solution if access and underuse of existing therapeutics remain problems.

As noted previously with the NIH funding assessment, aggregate disease categories could obscure what is happening for specific diseases. Taking neoplasms for example, some types of cancer could be driving the large investment numbers while others are relatively neglected. A breakdown by cancer type shows significant variation (Figure 3-5). According to this analysis, cancers with underinvestment relative to projected burden include tracheal, bronchus, and lung, as well as colon, rectum, and prostate. Even this more detailed assessment is limited because it does not further

---

[5] Lim et al., forthcoming.

72

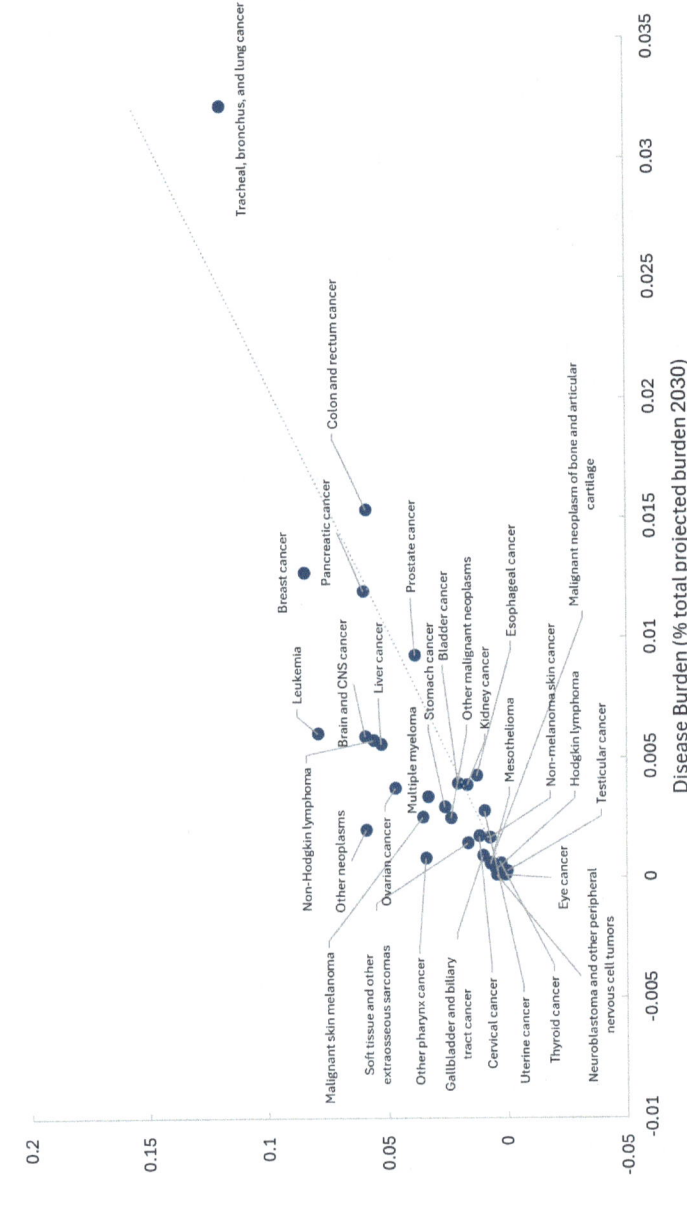

FIGURE 3-5 Comparison of total pipeline drugs versus proportion of U.S. DALYs for neoplasm subtypes projected in 2030. SOURCE: Adapted from IHME data.

disaggregate by cancer stage, nor does it include data that are not publicly available from small biotech companies, larger pharmaceutical corporations, or foundations. Other studies have shown underinvestment in early-stage cancer treatments and preventatives (Budish et al., 2015).

Comparing Private and Public Investment

Similar to the case with the NIH funding assessment, these data indicate substantial investment in HIV/AIDS and neurological disorders and under-investment in cardiovascular disease relative to burden. There is more private than public investment in skin and subcutaneous diseases and greater public investment in mental health disorders. Cancers, including prostate, colon and rectum, and lung, have fewer pipeline drugs but have approximately proportional NIH funding. This could indicate that public and private investment are complementary in these disease areas, or that there is a component of degree of scientific knowledge to develop compounds for the different diseases. Of note, comparisons between private and public investments are difficult to carry out, given that the analyses of these investments use both different metrics for investment (the number of products in the development pipeline for private investment versus federal support in dollars for public investment) and different disease categories. For example, IHME private-sector assessment uses 22 categories, while the NIH funding analysis includes 59.

Limitations of Data Available on Private-Sector Investment

In general, it is challenging to assess private-sector investment because of the lack of accessible data. For-profit companies are not incentivized to be forthcoming about the underlying financial details for their investments, and it is difficult to get a sense of what developments are early in the pipeline. It is also a dynamic space that can change rapidly, as with a new discovery. Not only is it hard to predict how the landscape of therapeutic development will change by 2030, but it is also difficult to tell from these data which gaps are related to unmet need versus market forces or other drivers.

Given these challenges, assessments of private investment typically use proxies, such as the number of products, patents, or clinical trials, to assess current and projected relative investments, but these data do not give a full understanding of where companies are directing their efforts. The IHME data described above rely on the availability of information on the number of pipeline pharmaceutical products and their uses. As these say nothing about the dollar amounts invested, the data cannot be directly compared with or combined with the NIH funding assessment or other analyses. These data also do not include products already on the market, which could provide insight into the dimension of unmet need or how past investments have contributed to the current landscape of available therapies. It is possible that some therapeutic areas with fewer products in the development pipeline have effective on-market treatments that are not accounted for in this cross-sectional analysis. Longitudinal data on investment trends would be helpful for addressing this limitation. In addition, this dataset includes information on all pharmaceutical companies at the time of analysis, including companies outside the United States, so some of these products do not reflect U.S. investment and may not be made for the U.S. market. Additional, more specific data would be useful to develop a more comprehensive picture of private-sector investment.

> Finding 3-1: Characterizing past, current, and future priorities for investments in therapeutic innovation is multidimensional and complicated, especially given the longitudinal nature of research and development. Many of the data needed for this purpose are not publicly available. Some high-level data on industry investment are available, but the granularity of this information is limited.

ADDITIONAL FACTORS TO CONSIDER

Disease burden encompasses multiple dimensions, including both population-level and individual-level impact (see Chapter 2). Considering individual burden draws attention to the significant unmet medical need in rare diseases—conditions that have low prevalence but high individual burden and for which there are often no effective treatments. A rare disease, by definition, affects fewer than 200,000 people in the United States, but in the aggregate, these conditions affect more than 30 million people in the United States (FDA, 2024). Of an estimated 7,000–10,000 rare diseases, only 5 percent have FDA-approved treatments, and many of these disorders are life threatening (Fermaglich and Miller, 2023).

Several other important factors could be overlooked in the data-driven approaches to assessing mismatch and prioritizing investment that have been described thus far in this chapter. Some conditions could be underrepresented or absent in these datasets, such as disease areas where there is contested diagnosis, a lack of effective diagnostics, or limited information (Adams et al., 2024). In addition, unmet need, one of this committee's focal points, is difficult to quantify when compared with burden or investment metrics. In some cases, therapeutic gaps persist because of the complexity of the underlying biology or gaps in scientific knowledge (Elmore et al., 2021). As discussed in more detail in Chapter 2, unmet need can exist because of a lack of effective therapeutics as well as a lack of health care access.

Health equity is another important factor to consider. Health disparities persist among racial and ethnic groups for many conditions in the United States (IOM, 2003; NASEM, 2024), as well as across other demographics, including rural/urban, age, and gender. While a condition may have existing therapeutic options, there may be unaddressed need if some groups do not have access to them. As another example, many therapies remain inaccessible to populations outside of urban medical centers, and investment in novel treatments or delivery mechanisms could address unmet need and improve health for some underserved groups and conditions. (NASEM, 2018).

Current approaches for assessing mismatch typically focus on the resulting diseases, but therapeutic targets could also include upstream risk factors such as obesity or smoking. Risk factors could be another lens through which to assess mismatch or identify areas for innovation. Lastly, a comprehensive assessment of mismatch between investment and burden should incorporate a future-oriented perspective, especially regarding up and coming technologies where innovative approaches can have significant effect.

PRIORITIZATION METHODS IN THE LITERATURE

Difficult decisions have to be made to prioritize among many competing therapeutic areas with high unmet need. There are a number of different approaches to research priority setting that vary in how they incorporate evaluation criteria, weight different normative values, and involve stakeholders. Millum (2024) provides a useful review of specific methods in the literature. Millum emphasizes that there is largely consensus on the two main objectives of research priority setting—maximizing population health benefits and improving equitable distribution of those benefits. However, there is disagreement in the literature over more detailed questions and process criteria. Importantly, how a research priority setting exercise is conducted, and who is involved, will shape outcomes, which could have important ethical implications (Millum, 2024). Those setting research priorities often account in some way for the relative level of disease burden and unmet need. In addition, some argue that projected burden for future populations should also be taken into account (Pierson, 2024).

Recognizing the complexities of assessing alignment among investment, burden, and unmet need, several groups have developed methods for prioritizing investment across various disease areas; a few examples follow. The Child Health and Nutrition Research Initiative's method involves a survey of a large number of experts, a set of criteria to rank their research priorities, and, depending on the goal of the selection, potentially involving funders or government bodies in the process (Millum, 2024). The Essential Health National Research Strategy—designed by the Council on Health Research and Development—convenes a national workshop of stakeholders (e.g., researchers, health service providers, private-sector professionals, potential donors). The working group then conducts a "situational analysis" to determine an initial list of research ideas that are later ranked based on a set of criteria and a scoring method agreed upon by the group (Millum, 2024).

The Milken Institute's FasterCures worked with representatives from the Centers for Disease Control and Prevention, NIH, FDA, the Office of the Assistant Secretary for Health, and others to develop a quantitative framework to identify and prioritize opportunities in biomedical product innovation. Gressler and colleagues (2023) selected a pilot list of 13 disease conditions based on the highest mortality, prevalence, and years lived with disability metrics. For each disease, the authors calculated the overall gap of innovation by using a public health burden score, health care cost score, and biomedical product innovation score—each score comprising multiple metrics (Gressler et al., 2023). This process identified diabetes, osteoarthritis, and drug use disorders as having the highest overall gap score. In addition, conditions with the lowest innovation despite significant burden included such chronic conditions as chronic kidney disease, chronic obstructive pulmonary disease, and cirrhosis and other liver diseases. The analysis sought to bring together multiple metrics to assess not only burden but also health care cost, public investment, and private investment (Gressler et al., 2023). This committee's statement of task does not include an assessment of health care cost and access, but the multifaceted approach could prove a useful example for future analysis as well.

The World Health Organization's (WHO's) foundational 1996 Ad Hoc Committee on Health Research Relating to Future Intervention Options developed a research prioritization method by convening technical experts to consider five questions regarding a health problem and assess its research gaps (WHO, 1996). The committee adapted this model to create a list of questions relevant to the statement of task's focus on U.S. disease burden and unmet need (Table 3-1). These questions may be helpful for assessing mismatch and priority setting, although data may not be readily available for all of these considerations.

CHAPTER CONCLUSION

This chapter reviewed evidence on how well public and private investment in therapeutic development align with disease burden and unmet need. The committee found:

Finding 3-2: There are some existing data on disease burden, unmet need, and investment; however, these data are not regularly compiled and synthesized for assessing mismatch across factors. In addition, existing data are sometimes insufficient and have significant gaps. As a

TABLE 3-1 Questions to Inform Research Priority Setting

WHO, 1996. 5-Step Process to Inform R&D Resource Allocation	Key Questions Adapted for This Report
Step 1: How big is the health problem? Calculate the burden attributable to the disease, condition, or risk factor. Step 2: Why does the disease burden persist? Identify reasons for the persistence of the burden of the disease or condition in a population. Step 3: Is enough known about the problem now to consider possible interventions? Judge the adequacy of the current knowledge base. Step 4: How cost-effective will these interventions be?[a] Assess the promise of the R&D effort. Step 5: How much is already being done about the problem? Assess the current level of effort.	What is the burden of disease based on occurrence (incidence, prevalence, severity, duration) and impact (on quality of life, economically on an individual, on caregivers, society, etc.)? How is it measured (e.g., DALYs)? Consider how population burden and impact may vary (e.g., high prevalence/moderate impact; low prevalence/high impact). What is the level and type of unmet need? For example: • No effective treatment • Treatment exists but is of limited effectiveness (overall or for targeted subgroups of population) • Treatment is effective, but access is limited (overall or for targeted subgroups of population) What is the current level of investment, and does it address the level of burden and unmet need? What are the barriers or challenges to innovation in therapeutic development for this therapeutic area (e.g., scientific challenges, market forces)?[b] What are potential strategies to spur innovation?[c]

[a] This committee's statement of task did not include assessment of cost-effectiveness.

[b] See the committee's discussion of barriers driving mismatch in Chapter 4.

[c] See Chapter 5 for a discussion of strategies and Chapter 6 for this committee's recommendations.

SOURCE: Parts of this table are adapted from Box S-2 in WHO, 1996. © Copyright World Health Organization (WHO), 2021. All Rights Reserved.

result, this committee lacked the data needed to produce a report that evaluates all aspects of disease burden, unmet need, and investment to fully assess the mismatch.

Taken together, the evidence suggests underinvestment relative to burden in some chronic conditions such as cardiovascular disease and

COPD. The committee's analysis of NIH funding versus disease burden (DALYs rate) also highlighted lower public investment in such conditions as headaches, neck and back pain, psoriasis, and gallbladder diseases. The sources on private-sector investment, though limited, indicate substantial investment in oncology and neurological disease and suggest underinvestment in cardiovascular disease and maternal and neonatal conditions. The following chapter will take a closer look at specific drivers that contribute to mismatches among investment, burden, and unmet need.

The analysis in this chapter reinforces the claim that the metrics and methodology used make a difference in which conditions appear most underinvested, emphasizing the need for a systematic, multifaceted assessment. As discussed, there are a number of limitations to the data available for this purpose. These limitations make it challenging to draw firm conclusions about mismatch and investment and underscore the need for better data and tracking. Moreover, no systematic, comprehensive reporting regularly occurs on the alignment between burden and investment. A commitment to regular collation and synthesis of data and to regular updating and reporting would help create a public good that is foundational to the goal of improving alignment between investments in innovation and unmet need. Furthermore, if public resources are used to collect this data, it is important that these data be made public, to the extent possible, to inform public health research. The use of public resources obligates the government to provide these data in a timely manner and reduce barriers to data access. A robust, timely, publicly accessible data system is key to implementing recommended changes in policies and practice that can deliver better health outcomes from the resources invested in innovation. Accordingly, the committee concludes:

Conclusion 3-1: More comprehensive, specific, timely, and accurate data on disease burden, unmet need, and innovation, as well as improved data aggregation, are essential for private and public funders to systematically use measures of disease burden and unmet need when making decisions about funding priorities.

Conclusion 3-2: Collecting and aggregating these data requires ongoing stewardship to most effectively address unmet clinical need and reduce health disparities.

Conclusion 3-3: The U.S. government has a responsibility to ensure that timely data on public investment and population health data be made publicly available to support research and strategic investment in areas of unmet need.

REFERENCES

Adams, D. R., C. D. M. van Karnebeek, S. B. Agulló, V. Faùndes, S. S. Jamuar, S. A. Lynch, G. Pintos-Morell, R. D. Puri, R. Shai, C. A. Steward, B. Tumiene, and A. Verloes. 2024. Addressing diagnostic gaps and priorities of the global rare diseases community: Recommendations from the IRDiRC Diagnostics Scientific Committee. *European Journal of Medical Genetics* 70:104951.

Ballreich, J. M., C. P. Gross, N. R. Powe, and G. F. Anderson. 2021. Allocation of National Institutes of Health funding by disease category in 2008 and 2019. *JAMA Network Open* 4(1):e2034890.

Best, R. K. 2012. Disease politics and medical research funding. *American Sociological Review* 77(5):780–803.

Budish, E., B. N. Roin, and H. Williams. 2015. Do firms underinvest in long-term research? Evidence from cancer clinical trials. *American Economic Review* 105(7):2044–2085.

Congressional Research Service. 2023. *National Institutes of Health (NIH) funding: FY1996-FY2023, updated March 8, 2023*. https://crsreports.congress.gov/product/pdf/R/R43341/45 (accessed April 13, 2025).

Congressional Research Service. 2024. *National Institutes of Health (NIH) Funding: FY1996-FY2025*. https://www.congress.gov/crs-product/R43341 (accessed May 21, 2025).

Ehrhardt, S., L. J. Appel, and C. L. Meinert. 2015. Trends in National Institutes of Health funding for clinical trials registered in ClinicalTrials.Gov. *JAMA* 314(23):2566.

Elmore, L. W., S. F. Greer, E. C. Daniels, C. C. Saxe, M. H. Melner, G. M. Krawiec, W. G. Cance, and W. C. Phelps. 2021. Blueprint for cancer research: Critical gaps and opportunities. *CA: A Cancer Journal for Clinicians* 71(2):107–139.

Fermaglich, L. J., and K. L. Miller. 2023. A comprehensive study of the rare diseases and conditions targeted by orphan drug designations and approvals over the forty years of the Orphan Drug Act. *Orphanet Journal of Rare Diseases* 18(1):163.

FDA (Food and Drug Administration). 2024. *Rare diseases at the FDA*. https://www.fda.gov/patients/rare-diseases-fda (accessed March 20, 2025).

FDA. 2025. *Advancing health through innovation: New drug therapy approvals 2024*. https://www.fda.gov/drugs/novel-drug-approvals-fda/novel-drug-approvals-2024 (accessed May 15, 2025).

Galkina Cleary, E., J. M. Beierlein, N. S. Khanuja, L. M. McNamee, and F. D. Ledley. 2018. Contribution of NIH funding to new drug approvals 2010-2016. *Proceedings of the National Academy of Sciences* 115(10):2329–2334.

Galkina Cleary, E., M. J. Jackson, E. W. Zhou, and F. D. Ledley. 2023. Comparison of research spending on new drug approvals by the National Institutes of Health vs. the pharmaceutical industry, 2010 2019. *JAMA Health Forum* 4(4):c230511.

Gandjour, A. 2024. Inclusion of phase III clinical trial costs in health economic evaluations. *BMC Health Services Research* 24(1):1158.

Gillum, L. A., C. Gouveia, E. R. Dorsey, M. Pletcher, C. D. Mathers, C. E. McCulloch, and S. C. Johnston. 2011. NIH disease funding levels and burden of disease. *PLoS ONE* 6(2):e16837.

Gressler, L. E., K. Crowley, E. Berliner, H. Leroy, E. Krofah, B. Eloff, D. Marinac-Dabic, and M. Vythilingam. 2023. A quantitative framework to identify and prioritize opportunities in biomedical product innovation: A proof-of-concept study. *JAMA Health Forum* 4(5):e230894.

Gupta, R. S., C. M. Warren, B. M. Smith, J. Jiang, J. A. Blumenstock, M. M. Davis, R. P. Schleimer, and K. C. Nadeau. 2019. Prevalence and severity of food allergies among US adults. *JAMA Network Open* 2(1):e185630.

IOM (Institute of Medicine). 2003. *Unequal treatment: Confronting racial and ethnic disparities in health care.* Washington, DC: The National Academies Press.

IQVIA. 2023. *Global trends in R&D 2023: Activity, productivity, and enablers.* IQVIA Institute for Human Data Science. https://www.iqvia.com/insights/the-iqvia-institute/reports-and-publications/reports/global-trends-in-r-and-d-2023 (accessed April 13, 2025).

IQVIA. 2025. *Proliferation of innovation over time.* IQVIA Institute for Human Data Science. https://www.iqvia.com/insights/the-iqvia-institute/reports-and-publications/reports/proliferation-of-innovation-over-time (accessed April 13, 2025).

Kang, S.-Y., M. Liu, J. Ballreich, R. Gupta, and G. Anderson. 2024. Biopharmaceutical pipeline funded by venture capital firms, 2014 to 2024. *Health Affairs Scholar* 2(10):qxae124.

Kassir, Z., A. Sarpatwari, B. Kocak, C. C. Kuza, and W. F. Gellad. 2020. Sponsorship and funding for gene therapy trials in the United States. *JAMA* 323(9):890.

Kantarjian, H. M., T. Fojo, M. Mathisen, and L. A. Zwelling. 2013. Cancer drugs in the United States: Justum pretium—the just price. *Journal of Clinical Oncology* 31(28):3600–3604.

Kocher, R., and B. Roberts. 2014. The calculus of cures. *New England Journal of Medicine* 370(16):1473–1475.

Light, D. W., and R. Warburton. 2011. Demythologizing the high costs of pharmaceutical research. *BioSocieties* 6(1):34–50.

Millum, J. 2024. Ethics and health research priority setting: A narrative review [version 1; peer review: 2 approved]. *Wellcome Open Research* 9:203.

Moses, H., III, D. H. M. Matheson, S. Cairns-Smith, B. P. George, C. Palisch, and E. R. Dorsey. 2015. The anatomy of medical research: US and international comparisons. *JAMA* 313(2):174–189.

NASEM (National Academies of Sciences, Engineering, and Medicine). 2018. 2. Factors That Affect Health-Care Utilization. In *Health-care utilization as a proxy in disability determination.* Washington, DC: The National Academies Press. Pp. 21-38

NASEM. 2024. *Unequal treatment revisited: The current state of racial and ethnic disparities in health care: Proceedings of a workshop.* Washington, DC: The National Academies Press.

NCI (National Cancer Institute). n.d. *Cancer facts & the war on cancer.* https://training.seer.cancer.gov/disease/war/ (accessed March 18, 2025).

NIH (National Institutes of Health). 2023. *Background—NIH peer review process.* https://grants.nih.gov/policy/peer/simplifying-review/background.htm (accessed April 13, 2025).

NIH. 2024. *Mission and goals.* https://www.nih.gov/about-nih/what-we-do/mission-goals (accessed May 21, 2025).

NIH RePORT (Research Portfolio and Online Reporting Tools). n.d. *RCDC: Categorization process.* https://report.nih.gov/funding/categorical-spending/rcdc-process (accessed May 21, 2025).

Ouellette, L. L., and B. N. Sampat. 2024. Using Bayh-Dole Act march-in rights to lower US drug prices. *JAMA Health Forum* 5(11):e243775.

OMB (Office of Management and Budget). 2025. *Letter to Susan Collins, chair of the Committee on Appropriations.* https://www.whitehouse.gov/wp-content/uploads/2025/05/Fiscal-Year-2026-Discretionary-Budget-Request.pdf (accessed May 30, 2025).

Pierson, L. 2024. Accounting for future populations in health research. *Bioethics* 38(5):401–409.

Rees, C. A., M. C. Monuteaux, V. Herdell, E. W. Fleegler, and F. T. Bourgeois. 2021. Correlation between National Institutes of Health funding for pediatric research and pediatric disease burden in the US. *JAMA Pediatrics* 175(12):1236.

Rome, B. N., A. S. Kesselheim, and W. B. Feldman. 2024. Medicare's first round of drug-price negotiation—Measuring success. *New England Journal of Medicine* 391(20):1865–1868.

Sansweet, S., C. Rolling, M. Ebisawa, J. Wang, R. Gupta, and C. M. Davis. 2024. Reaching communities through food allergy advocacy, research, and education: A comprehensive analysis. *Journal of Allergy and Clinical Immunology: In Practice* 12(2):310–315.

SiRM (Strategies in Regulated Markets), L.E.K. Consulting, and RAND Europe. 2022. *The financial ecosystem of pharmaceutical R&D: An evidence base to inform further dialogue.* https://www.rand.org/content/dam/rand/pubs/external_publications/EP60000/EP68954/RAND_EP68954.pdf (accessed May 30, 2025).

Stoelinga, J., L. T. Bloem, M. Russo, A. S. Kesselheim, and W. B. Feldman. 2024. Comparing supplemental indications for cancer drugs approved in the U.S. and EU. *European Journal of Cancer* 212:114330.

Wang, D., B. Liu, and Z. Zhang. 2023. Accelerating the understanding of cancer biology through the lens of genomics. *Cell* 186(8):1755–1771.

WHO (World Health Organization). 1996. *Investing in health research and development: Report of the Ad Hoc Committee on Health Research Relating to Future Intervention Options.* Geneva, Switzerland: World Health Organization. https://iris.who.int/handle/10665/63024 (accessed April 13, 2025).

4

Factors Contributing to
Misalignment Between
Investment Priorities and Unmet Need

The idea of accelerating medical breakthroughs and enabling individualized screening, prevention, treatments, and care for all depends on appropriately integrated funding for science, clinical trials, and data aggregation and analysis, as well as regulatory considerations. Barriers in any one of these areas impede innovation. Although there are many challenges and barriers in drug development broadly, this chapter seeks to narrowly focus on the reasons underlying the observed mismatch between research and development investments and areas of unmet need. Exemplars are used throughout to highlight disease areas where innovations are not meeting patients' needs because of these barriers.

SCIENTIFIC CHALLENGES

Lack of Understanding of Underlying Pathophysiology

One of the factors driving a misalignment of investment with disease burden and unmet need is a lack of understanding of the underlying pathophysiology of certain diseases. Public funding for basic and translational research is critical for understanding the basic mechanisms of disease and thus for developing potential molecular targets for drug discovery and development (see Chapter 3). As explained by Tal Zaks, Partner at OrbiMed, former chief medical officer at Moderna, and an oncologist by training, during an open session for this report, "Our starting point [as an investor] is not unmet need nor disease burden; rather, our starting point is something new that gives us the opportunity to do something about it."[1] Private innovation and commercialization of therapeutics that improve outcomes of patients is inextricably linked to public investment in biomedical research (discussed further in Chapter 5).

However, there are some disease areas reviewed in Chapter 3 that continue to receive fewer research dollars from the National Institutes of Health (NIH) despite large unmet needs. Chronic obstructive pulmonary disease (COPD), for example, affects approximately 11.7 million adults in the United States and costs around $50 billion annually (American Lung Association, 2024a), but it receives relatively low public investment for research (Chapter 3), and little progress has been made on new innovative targets for COPD patients (Barnes et al., 2015). COPD is a heterogeneous condition, including chronic bronchitis and emphysema, characterized by a variety of respiratory symptoms and smoking history (American Lung Association, 2024b). Because of the heterogeneity of the disease, it is difficult to develop a one-size-fits-all approach to therapeutic development for COPD (Leung et al., 2019). More investment into developing a precision-medicine approach or developing better animal models could help improve innovation and the development of therapeutic targets for COPD (Barnes et al., 2015; Leung et al., 2019).

There are certain disease areas, such as neurodegenerative disorders, where research investments are high and where those investments may be warranted, given the levels of disease burden and unmet needs. However, despite these high levels of investments, innovation has not yet been able to meet the needs of many patients. Box 4-1 describes one of these examples, Alzheimer's disease (AD), in more detail. The committee emphasizes that even in areas where there is a strong public commitment to investment, the complexity of some diseases results in significant residual unmet need, leading to fewer molecular drug targets that researchers can use to pursue therapeutic discovery and development. Furthermore, when potential molecular targets are identified, such as for AD, the lack of a detailed understanding of the pathophysiology and disease progression deters investment in moving such molecular targets forward owing to the uncertainty in whether the target will ultimately lead to an innovative, disease-modifying therapeutic. Thus, identifying validated molecular targets for drug development is a key consideration. This may also include needing novel diagnostic tests to characterize disease and disease states and to better identify patients who should receive novel treatments, as described in Box 4-1.

Although there are still many areas where a lack of understanding of the disease mechanism results in a large unmet need, there are new technologies

---

[1] T. Zaks and M. Mackay. 2024. *Strategies to better align investments in innovations for therapeutic development with disease burden and unmet needs.* Meeting 2, June 18, 2024.

BOX 4-1
Therapeutic Development for Alzheimer's Disease

Alzheimer's disease (AD) is a progressive neurodegenerative disorder that is one of the leading causes of death in the United States (Kochanek et al., 2022). It is estimated that 6.9 million individuals in the United States are living with AD, and that number is expected to nearly double by the year 2050 (Alzheimer's Association, 2024). AD is also a correspondingly costly disease, with its estimated annual cost to the U.S. economy in 2010 around $307 billion (Zissimopoulos et al., 2014). This annual cost is anticipated to rise significantly to $1.5 trillion by 2050, as the population ages and caregiving and related health care costs increase. It is estimated that innovation in drug discovery that could delay onset of AD by even 5 years would drastically reduce the cost per person and would extend both life-years and quality of life for those living with AD and their caregivers.

Unmet Need

Despite its high prevalence and cost, there are relatively few approved treatments for AD. Currently, a total of eight drugs on the market have been approved for the treatment of AD: six medications to treat the symptoms of dementia and two that marginally delay disease progression (Alzheimer's Association, 2024). The two drugs that alter disease progression (lecanemab and donanemab) are monoclonal antibodies that can be prescribed to patients with mild cognitive impairment. Though the evidence on the relationship between amyloid-beta and clinical outcomes is inconclusive (Ackley et al., 2021; Pang et al., 2023), these drugs target either soluble oligomeric forms of the protein, amyloid-beta, in the case of lecanemab, or insoluble aggregated, deposited plaques of amyloid-beta, which is the mechanism of action for donanemab. Therefore, confirmation of amyloid plaques in the brain is required prior to initiating treatment. These medications both lead to small improvements in cognitive and functional measures which, despite being statistically significant, fall below the minimal clinically important difference, which means that the difference may not be observable by patients or caregivers (ICER, 2023). Despite excitement about these medications, the small magnitude of their clinical benefit and the substantial risks associated with their use limits their value for many patients.

First, both medications contain a boxed warning for amyloid-related imaging abnormalities (ARIAs), which often present as temporary brain swelling that may be accompanied by small brain bleeds (FDA, 2023, 2024a). Although ARIAs are usually asymptomatic, they can be accom-

continued

BOX 4-1 Continued

panied by serious intracerebral hemorrhages and neurologic deficits. Three people enrolled in the lecanemab study died during the extended phase of the trial because of complications such as brain bleeding or seizures, which may have been caused by ARIA (Piller, 2022). Second, strict eligibility criteria for the clinical trials for these medications may mean that they will show reduced efficacy when used by a broader patient population, which often has comorbidities and mixed pathologies (Walsh et al., 2022). Finally, these medications are expensive, which greatly limits their accessibility. For example, lecanemab costs $26,500 annually, exclusive of the frequent brain scans, tests, and monitoring required for safe use.

Barriers to Innovation and Therapeutic Development

Despite the high disease burden and the unmet need of safe and effective therapies for AD, more significant innovation for AD treatment remains a challenging and perhaps elusive goal. This cannot be attributed to a lack of investment, as the National Institutes of Health is spending around $3.8 billion annually on AD-related research, and it is estimated that industry spent roughly $42.5 billion in AD research in development between 1995 and 2021 (Alzheimer's Association, n.d.; Cummings et al., 2022). However, it may be that investment is not ocused on the most promising scientific areas. For example, while the amyloid hypothesis has been the dominant explanation for Alzheimer's, it has also been controversial, and not all researchers accept it (Begley, 2019; Selkoe, 2025).

Another potential reason for the shortfall in therapeutic development may be related to inadequate innovation in AD diagnostics. It is costly and time consuming for many patients to receive a diagnosis of mild cognitive impairment and to undergo scans to confirm the presence of beta-amyloid plaques to qualify for the likely more optimal earlier administration of one of these disease-modifying medications. Furthermore, evaluating the changes in cognition that result in quality-of-life improvements remains a challenge. New innovations in diagnostics, such as a new blood test for amyloid plaques, which was cleared by the Food and Drug Administration for marketing in May 2025 could help diagnose patients earlier in the disease progression and be minimally invasive (Ashton et al., 2024; FDA, 2025). It is possible, that with earlier intervention, the efficacy of these agents may be enhanced.

Another advancement that could spur innovation is to improve the availability of newer, druggable targets for slowing or modifying AD progression. As artificial intelligence (AI) and deep learning models improve

BOX 4-1 Continued

and are used more frequently in biomedical research, they could help identify such new targets for drug discovery and development (Zhang et al., 2023). For example, a 2019 study used deep learning to scan the PubChem compound library to identify potential inhibitors for the peptide primarily found in beta-amyloid plaques associated with AD (Kaushik et al., 2019).

Until there are better drug targets, improved diagnostics, and more affordable and accessible medication options for patients, AD will remain an area of high disease burden with a large unmet need for therapeutics options.

---

that could be potentially transformative and lead to more productive drug discovery efforts in these areas. For example, artificial intelligence (AI) has the potential to transform drug discovery by identifying novel targets and to improve safety by predicting toxicological patterns as well as exploiting other actionable insights (Paul et al., 2021). AI can help in understanding the basic mechanisms of disease and could be transformative for the current system. However, the committee acknowledges that there are several limitations and challenges to using AI in drug development, including data-quality issues that compromise accuracy, concerns with black-box models producing incorrect or misleading results, and trust issues among patients and trial participants, particularly related to accessing patient datasets, which would be critical for training and validation of AI algorithms (Paul et al., 2021).

Advances in platform technologies is another area that could play a critical role in therapeutic innovation. Platforms represent highly versatile approaches for developing innovative therapeutics, which are to varying degrees independent of molecular targets. Examples of platform technologies include viral vectors for gene therapy, CRISPR for gene editing, small interfering RNAs, antisense oligonucleotide technologies, structure-based drug design, mRNA therapeutics, and intracellular targeted protein degradative platforms. PROTACs monoclonal antibodies are one example of an intracellular targeted protein degradative platform, which includes libraries for screening and discovery of novel agents that selectively bind to targets. These platform technologies can also expedite drug development by not having to be validated every time they are used, and the Food and Drug Administration (FDA) has published guidance to help clarify how to request platform technology designation (Niazi, 2024).

As these technologies are developed, they can become the basis for start-up companies or be licensed to existing or larger biopharmaceutical companies for the use in discovery and development of new agents. The development of platform technologies has enabled scientific advances such as gene cloning, recombinant production of proteins, gene sequencing, and the discovery and early development of monoclonal antibodies. As advances in platform technologies continue, so will our understanding of diseases and the development of treatments to address them.

Finding 4-1: Investment in basic and preclinical biomedical research is essential to driving innovation in disease areas with significant disease burden that have unmet needs.

Challenges Measuring Outcomes

Difficulty measuring health outcomes can drive mismatches between investment and unmet need in some disease areas. When outcomes are subjective, hard to characterize, or highly variable, companies may face higher development costs, risk, and uncertainty, which can lead them to direct resources toward other disease areas where outcomes are better established and more easily measured. Many conditions lack objective biomarkers that could help characterize the disease more precisely and provide early signals of treatment efficacy, thereby derisking investment and accelerating drug development.

Chronic pain is a prototypical example of this type of challenge (see Box 4-2 for more detail). Inherently subjective, pain generally lacks objective outcome measures or biomarkers, so physicians and researchers must rely on patient-reported scales, which are subject to variability, in order to evaluate patients' complex pain symptoms (Dansie and Turk, 2013; Robinson-Papp et al., 2015). Although these subjective measures are important, they often create noisy datasets, which make it more challenging to receive FDA approval. Similarly, psychiatric disorders such as depression rely heavily on symptom reporting via questionnaires and have limited biomarkers or objective indicators that can be measured reliably (Abi-Dargham et al., 2023; Levis et al., 2019). In fibromyalgia, widespread musculoskeletal pain, fatigue, stiffness, and cognitive difficulties manifest without clear underlying tissue damage or reliable diagnostic biomarkers (Favretti et al., 2023). Other conditions characterized by functional impairments rather than by clear physiological problems, such as irritable bowel syndrome, and those diagnosed clinically by exclusion, such as chronic fatigue syndrome, further illustrate this challenge. The lack of established biomarkers or surrogate endpoints that reliably correspond to clinical benefit makes drug development more complicated and

BOX 4-2
Challenges in Therapeutic Development for Chronic Pain

It is estimated that 51.6 million Americans live with chronic pain (Rikard et al., 2023). Pain is considered chronic when it persists for more than 3 months, but chronic pain can persist for years or even a lifetime, with major effects on quality of life (Rikard et al., 2023). Chronic pain varies in sensation, in severity, and in cause. For some, pain is caused by injury or accident, while others experience chronic pain because of an underlying disease, such as fibromyalgia.

Unmet Need

Because pain is unique for every person, it is difficult to develop effective treatments, and the general approach to pain management is to treat the pain itself, not the underlying cause of the pain. Furthermore, pain is variable over time, with some patients experiencing pain at certain times of the day. This may be explained by social phenomena (i.e., less activity and distraction later in the day) or by changes in circadian rhythms (NASEM, 2018). Treatment for pain is usually multidisciplinary, and may involve medications, physical therapy, diet and nutrition, meditation, interventional procedures, and more (Staudt, 2022). However, these team-based approaches lead to challenges for patients, including poor reimbursement for these services and a limited number of multidisciplinary clinics (Staudt, 2022).

Pharmacologic treatment of pain is one of the oldest approaches to treating pain, but with a checkered past (Paladini et al., 2023). Medications for pain management are typically divided into two categories: nonopioid analgesic agents and opioid analgesic agents. Opioid analgesics are effective in treating both chronic and acute pain (Cohen et al., 2025). However, opioids have a high risk for misuse, especially when prescribed for chronic pain, which can lead to increased dependency, tolerance, and eventual addiction to opioids (Cohen et al., 2025). As the United States continues to struggle with an opioid epidemic, started in part by the widespread use of the opioid oxycodone for pain in the early 2000s, prescription guidelines for opioid analgesics have tightened. In 2016, the Centers for Disease Control and Prevention released guidelines for prescribing opioids "only if the expected benefits for both pain and function will outweigh risks to the patient" (Dowell et al., 2016, p. 1638).

A variety of nonopioid analgesics have received Food and Drug Administration (FDA) approval to treat pain with varying effectiveness for patients (Derry et al., 2016; Kingwell, 2025). However, many of these medications have been on the market for many years and do not provide

continued

BOX 4-2 Continued

adequate relief to patients, especially for chronic pain. Therefore, newer drug targets for nonopioid analgesics are needed to provide patients with relief.

Challenges to Innovation

There have been efforts to develop new nonopioid analgesics. However, these trials have faced a range of clinical development issues, including challenges showing efficacy for FDA approval. This is largely because data for pain trials are often noisy due to the individualized nature of pain and because efficacy is evaluated by subjective measures from patients rather than by an objective outcome measure. Even for nonopioid analgesics that do make it past the regulatory approval stage, insurers have been reluctant to cover these therapies, which are more expensive than generic opioids (Cohen, 2024).

Despite these barriers, some sponsors are continuing to support a portfolio of nonopioid analgesics. For example, one company has developed a master pain protocol, with which it hopes to coordinate trial sites so patients can be transferred easily between trials or drugs, rather than having to recruit a trial from scratch each time (Waldron, 2023). The National Institutes of Health (NIH) also has an NIH-wide effort to stem the opioid epidemic through its The Helping to End Addiction Long-term® Initiative, or NIH HEAL Initiative®, which includes developing a clinical research portfolio for pain management (NIH, 2024b).

---

uncertain, driving up costs and disincentivizing innovation in these areas of high unmet need.

MARKET FORCES

Bringing a new drug to market is an expensive and lengthy process. Only about 12 percent of drugs that enter phase I clinical trials ultimately demonstrate effectiveness and safety and thus are granted FDA approval (Congressional Budget Office, 2021). In 2021, the Congressional Budget Office reviewed three prior studies on pharmaceutical research and development (R&D) costs, which estimated the average cost to bring a new drug to market ranges from $0.8 billion to $2.3 billion (in 2019 dollars), including capital costs and the costs of failed investments (Congressional Budget Office, 2021). Two more recent studies reached similar estimates of approximately $900 million (in 2018 dollars) and $1.1 billion, also including the costs of capital and failures (Sertkaya et al., 2024; Wouters and Kesselheim, 2024).

As discussed in Chapter 1, since clinical trials are so expensive and lengthy and are often associated with a great deal of risk, they generally require substantial investments from for-profit entities, such as venture capital firms or drug companies, to complete. As these entities seek profits for their shareholders, concerns about returns on investment are of paramount importance for drug developers. Risk-adjusted net present value (NPV) forecasts are done for each project and drive investment decisions concerning which assets should continue through development, approval, and on to the market (or remain on market) and which assets should be shelved. NPV forecasts are used to analyze potential return on investment (Gallo, 2014), accounting for a number of factors, including the likely volume of usage, the net pricing of the envisioned product, and the duration of patent coverage or market exclusivity. Each of these considerations is complicated by such factors as the size of the target patient population, disease severity, associated diagnosis and treatment rates, presence or absence and relative attractiveness of existing competing products, willingness of payers to cover, degree of formulary coverage, and utilization management.

Some of these NPV drivers prevent drug developers from investing in therapeutics and diagnostics (see Box 4-3) because the potential return on investment from such a new therapy may be lower than their defined hurdle rate and thus does not justify further investment in research and development. For example, many drugs, particularly vaccines, have been shelved because of poor market prospects (Krishnamurthy et al., 2022). Acemoglu and Linn documented that innovation, measured as the number of new products entering the market, increased by 4–6 percent per 1 percent increase in the expected market size of a product (Acemoglu and Linn, 2004). This section reviews some of these market forces that drive misalignments in investments in innovation with disease burden and unmet need.

Patient Population Size

Traditionally, the ability of manufacturers to recover R&D investments is particularly limited for disease states with small patient populations. Rare diseases, as discussed earlier in the report, by definition affect small populations.[2] Current estimates indicate that about 30 million people have been diagnosed with a rare disease, also known as an orphan disease, and

---

[2] The Orphan Drug Act definition of rare disease also includes a disease that "affects more than 200,000 in the United States and for which there is no reasonable expectation that the cost of developing and making available in the United States a drug for such disease or condition will be recovered from sales in the United States of such drug." 21 U.S. Code § 360bb(a)(2).

BOX 4-3
Disincentives to Developing Diagnostics

Although diagnostics are critical for developing more effective thera-peutics, as discussed in Box 4-1, the attention and funding they receive has lagged behind therapeutic development. According to the former Food and Drug Administration (FDA) commissioner, Dr. Rob Califf, the innovation and creativity is there for diagnostics, but the limited progress in diagnostics is "as much an FDA issue as it is a payment issue."[a] The regulatory system and the payment system are interconnected, leading to a lack of investment in diagnostic tests.

On the regulatory side, diagnostics are regulated as medical devices, which is different from how drugs are regulated. Because medical de-vices encompass such a wide range of products, FDA sorts devices into three classes (class I, II, and III) depending on the controls needed to prove safety and efficacy.[b] Only class III products require premarket ap-proval before they can be sold.[c]

Many diagnostics on the market did not require premarket approval, which results in the presence of a variety of diagnostic tests of varying quality and efficacy. Companion diagnostics, which are diagnostics tied to the approval of a certain medication (for example, a genetic test to identify a mutation that a companion therapeutic targets) are regulated as class III products and therefore require premarket approval (FDA, 2014). Because these diagnostics are tied to use of a therapeutic, drug companies are motivated to validate the clinical significance of diagnos-tics (Eisenberg, 2019).

However, many diagnostic companies have begun to seek FDA ap-proval for class I or II devices, even though it is not legally necessary, because health insurers require FDA approval if they are to cover the cost of the testing (Eisenberg, 2019). This can result in a less efficient diagnostic approach. For example, insurers may cover a less compre-hensive genetic test that focuses only on clinically validated mutations shown to predict treatment response, rather than broader tests that may reveal unknown mutations, such as those that could be unveiled through next-generation sequencing, which may have treatment and research implications (Green Park Collaborative, 2015). Therefore, coverage deci-sions may restrict development of more comprehensive diagnostics that could be useful for identifying and developing innovative therapeutics for novel targets.

---

[a] Rob Califf, November 21, 2024.
[b] 21 U.S.C. § 360c et seq.
[c] 21 U.S.C. § 360c et seq.

that there are between 7,000 and potentially more than 10,000 distinct rare disease diagnoses (FDA, 2024b; Haendel et al., 2020).

Because rare diseases affect such small populations, the market for uptake of these therapies is small, and for many years the return on investment often was correspondingly too low for successful performance in the market. Most rare diseases are categorized as ultrarare and hyperrare diseases and may affect fewer than 100 people globally, making the market for these drugs extremely small (Vavassori et al., 2024).

The scientific complexity of conducting drug development research for rare diseases is also a significant barrier, again, related to the low disease prevalence, heterogenous populations, and challenges in recruiting patients, among other issues (Fonseca et al., 2019). Additionally, the current knowledge base for many of these diseases is severely lacking. For example, many rare genetic diseases have poorly understood or complex pathophysiological mechanisms, highly heterogeneous presentations of disease, inadequate diagnostic approaches, and limited information about disease progression, creating an initial barrier to drug development. Conducting initial clinical trials for these drugs is especially challenging because of the small pool of eligible patients who may also be geographically dispersed, a financial burden that deters investment in this area (Kempf et al., 2018). Clinical trials with small sample sizes may face significant statistical issues and may not capture adequate data related to safety or effectiveness (NASEM, 2024b).

To address these challenges, several regulatory and policy actions have been implemented, such as the passage of the Orphan Drug Act in 1983 (see Chapter 5 for a longer description of the Orphan Drug Act). The act was designed to promote R&D in this area through tax credits for biopharmaceutical companies, waivers of FDA user fees, and increases in marketing exclusivity for rare indications, among other actions (Yates and Hinkel, 2022). Still today, fewer than 5 percent of rare diseases have approved drugs on the market (NASEM, 2024b). The gap is larger for those rare diseases affecting bone and connective tissue, ophthalmic, renal, urinary, and reproductive systems (Fonseca et al., 2019).

Diseases with large patient populations may also present challenges to potential investments in innovative products. For one, generics may already be available on the market, limiting investors' expectations for their return on investment. Moreover, payers are less likely to be willing to pay high prices for drugs that would be used by a large segment of the population, to avoid large increases in insurance premiums. This too could discourage investment in products with potentially large patient populations.

Patient Access

In the United States, manufacturers set the list, or sticker, price for their products. Government agencies mandate certain rebates and discounts for the programs they manage (e.g., Medicaid and 340B), and private insurers negotiate for rebates with manufacturers for the programs they manage (e.g., commercial insurance and Medicare Part D). Manufacturers seek a profit-maximizing price, which is influenced by the relative competition within the drug class and pricing decisions of their competitors (Pauly, 2017). Manufacturers may mark prices up or down from benchmark prices, depending on how agents and their product profiles are projected to address the needs of patients for the particular indication, as well as their competitiveness in the marketplace. Payers then typically determine whether and how to cover, reimburse, and manage the use of the products. When there is no coverage for a product, there is typically less prescribing and patient filling of prescriptions since patients would be responsible for paying the undiscounted list price of the drug. Thus the commercial returns in the Unites States to drug manufacturers are directly tied to the list and net pricing and access for physicians and patients. Moreover, the U.S. market is the world's largest and generally accounts for over half of global product revenues and 64–78 percent of profits, making U.S. assumptions about pricing and access key drivers of investment decisions regarding drug development (ASPE, 2024; Goldman and Lakdawalla, 2018).

Formularies

One market force that limits innovation despite high disease burden and unmet need is the availability of less effective therapeutic options, particularly those without patent protection, in certain disease states. Some high-burden diseases, such as cardiovascular disease (discussed more below), have some treatment options available, but these therapeutics may not fully address the disease for many reasons. For example, the effectiveness of available therapies may be limited in their ability to control symptomatology and disease progression and, ultimately address the underlying etiology of the disease, resulting in residual unmet need for patients. Theoretically, if a new drug that was more effective than current treatments were approved by the FDA, it would seem from basic market principles that the new drug would generate enough profits to make the investment worthwhile. However, the formulary design process does not always allow for this to be the case.

Health insurers often subcontract the coverage and administration of drugs dispensed from pharmacies (outpatient pharmacy benefits) to pharmacy benefit managers (PBMs), which reimburse pharmacies for claims, create pharmacy networks, and also design formularies (Hernandez and Hung, 2024). Formularies are "lists of drug products covered by [health plans] that distinguish between preferred or discouraged products by dividing outpatient therapies into three to five 'tiers,' each with a different level of patient cost sharing" (Werble, 2017, p. 41). Formulary designs also often involve utilization management tools that restrict coverage by requiring prior authorization (approval by the plan before prescribing or filling the drug), or evidence that a lower-cost or preferred drug has not worked for the patient before obtaining the higher-cost, nonpreferred drug, often called "step therapy."

In the formulary-making process, PBMs negotiate with manufacturers to obtain lower prices (typically through rebates that are paid by manufacturers after the product is sold) in exchange for coverage, favorable cost sharing, and lower use of utilization management relative to any competitors (Dickson et al., 2023) (more on this in Chapter 5). These negotiations typically favor the PBMs when there are multiple drugs in a class, but not in cases where there are limited treatment options or where formulary coverage is required. For example, in Medicare Part D, all plans are required to cover essentially all drugs in six protected classes: anticonvulsants, antidepressants, antineoplastics (cancer drugs), antipsychotics, antiretrovirals, and immunosuppressants (Cubanski, 2024).

In other therapeutic classes, they must cover at least two FDA-approved drugs per class. PBMs thus have less negotiating leverage for drugs in protected classes or classes with little competition. For example, for antineoplastic drugs—a category of drugs that typically has high per-user prices owing to smaller populations treated—there is evidence that Medicare's coverage requirements lead to limited or no rebating (meaning the list price set by the manufacturer is close to the amount paid by the plans and patients (Hwang et al., 2022). The required formulary coverage and ability to command high prices and pay lower rebates is generally considered an incentive for development, which may explain why the committee found disproportionate investment relative to disease burden for antineoplastic drugs and significant investments in therapeutics for mental health disorders (Chapter 3).

Because PBMs have greater negotiating leverage in competitive drug classes, this can serve as a barrier to innovation in disease states where available therapeutic options are able to only partially address disease burden, thus leading to residual unmet need. One example where this happens is in therapeutics for cardiovascular disease. Because there are a wide range of products available that are effective for many but not all patients, there are few incentives to develop new therapeutics for cardiovascular disease that could address residual unmet need in this area. While not the only factor, this may explain why the committee found cardiovascular disease to be an area that is underinvested relative to disease burden, as described in Chapter 3. However, because cardiovascular disease affects so many people, this lack of innovation results in residual unmet needs for patients.

Variation in Coverage and Reimbursement Across Payers

There exists important variation in coverage and reimbursement across payers, which may introduce differential incentives for R&D investment. Private insurance accounts for the largest share of spending on drugs in the United States, at 42 percent, but Medicare is the largest single source of spending, accounting for 30 percent of U.S. expenditures on drugs (Cubanski et al., 2019). Following the enactment of Medicare Part D, R&D activity increased for drug products with a high share of the Medicare-eligible population (Blume-Kohout and Sood, 2013). The prices of drugs that are largely paid for by Medicaid are consistently lower than in Medicare and commercial insurance because of the Medicaid Drug Rebate Program, which requires manufacturers of branded products to provide a base discount of 23 percent off of the average manufacturer price or the best price provided in the market, in addition to an inflation rebate that penalizes increases in drug prices above inflation (Dolan, 2019). This reimbursement structure may lead to decreased revenues for manufacturers (Dolan et al., 2021), which may in turn discourage the development of products with a high share of Medicaid use.

The Inflation Reduction Act (IRA) of 2022 introduced important reforms to the reimbursement of drug products under Medicare (see Box 5-4 for more details).[3] In addition to introducing inflation penalties in Medicare, the IRA conferred authority to the Centers for Medicare & Medicaid Services (CMS) to directly negotiate prices with manufacturers for 10 to 20 drugs per year, with negotiated prices applied beginning in 2026. CMS draft guidance released in May 2025 acknowledges that unmet need is one of the factors to be considered in the negotiation process (Klomp, 2025).

Limited Applicability of Therapeutics in Terms of Treatment Duration or Circumstances

The duration of use of a therapy is also an important market force. For drug developers, there is a greater incentive to invest in chronic disease states where the duration of therapy is not limited and therefore, there are greater opportunities to recover research and development costs than with acute conditions. The reason this occurs is two-fold. One issue is described

---

[3] Inflation Reduction Act of 2022, H.R.5376, 117th Congress (2022), https://www.congress.gov/bill/117th-congress/house-bill/5376 (accessed May 31, 2025).

in the behavioral economics literature of irrational purchaser preferences. Although it is rational to pay a lot more up front to cure a disease than to make a steady stream of payments over time, there is a tendency to underestimate the true cost of the stream of payments. This is because of significant underestimation of future costs, known as hyperbolic discounting (Kirby, 1997), and because of underestimation of total cost when it is divided into separate payments, known as partitioned pricing (Greenleaf et al., 2016; Lee et al., 2014; Morwitz et al., 1998; Xue and Ouellette, 2020).

This is further complicated by the fragmented U.S. health insurance system, and specifically, by the "churn" in commercial insurance coverage. Since people change insurance plans so frequently in the United States, no single insurer wants to pay the large costs up front, since it may lose the patient to another plan shortly thereafter and not receive any long-term savings from their high short-term investment in treatment. Furthermore, states with balanced budget requirements (35 states require the budget to be balanced at year end) make it challenging for state programs, such as Medicaid, to pay such a large sum up front (Tax Policy Center Urban Institute & Brookings Institution, n.d.).

The second reason is that even if purchasers are totally rational, a company with market power (as a result of having a patented drug) will find producing a repeat-purchase product more profitable than a onetime cure, which is what economists would call a "durable good" (Bureau of Economic Analysis, 2018). A manufacturer may be happy to sell a durable good (in this case, a curative therapy) at a high price at first for patients willing to pay but will eventually want to lower the price in the future to elicit more sales from patients who were unwilling to pay the initially high price. This pricing strategy risks limiting sales if payers are unwilling or unable to make the budgetary adjustments necessary to ensure access to these products. Therefore, manufacturers may prefer to develop and commercialize a less durable good that would allow for lower pricing but longer-term use to achieve their desired profits.

The situation described above creates a disincentive to develop curative therapies that have short treatment times. Treatments for hepatitis C are an illustrative example of this problem. When the early direct-acting antiviral drugs and drug combinations became available, their pricing became problematic since a defined treatment course of several weeks led to a cure. Because there was no possibility of an "annuity" over time within which to recoup investment, there was a market reluctance to invest in successful products (as in the case of Sovaldi), along with the required investment in many of the other programs that often prove to be failures. When successful treatments were developed, the cost of those treatments became a major barrier to access because of the high per-patient costs and the number of eligible patients. In addition, many patients in need of treatment were covered under state budgets (including those incarcerated and those insured under state Medicaid programs), which meant that access to treatments varied by where a person lived.

While some payers eventually decided to cover the cost of these therapies because treating hepatitis C reduces its spread and ultimately reduces the target population of those needing treatment, the country is still far from the goal of eradicating hepatitis C (Fleurence and Collins, 2023). Although the landscape for coverage of these drugs is changing, only eight states have eliminated coverage restrictions that limit access to these drugs (Davey et al., 2024). Largely not factored into such health economic assessments was the potential for developing liver cancers over a longer period of time, which would not be a factor for commercial payers whose insured populations are typically only enrolled in their plans for relatively short periods of time, as described above. The commensurate reduction in cost burden to payers over time resulted in some additional coverage for these medications, although more coverage will be needed to eradicate hepatitis C.

> *Conclusion 4-1: Innovative therapies are emerging for rare diseases and other complex conditions, offering a potential for cure. However, the fragmented payment system within the United States is a barrier to patient access, resulting in underinvestment in developing curative therapies. The current U.S. market and policy environment is unprepared to manage these one-time, very high-cost therapies. There is a need for a clearer reimbursement structure for innovators developing these high-cost curative treatments.*

These same market forces can also apply to the development of drugs for exceptional (low-probability, high-risk) circumstances, such as countermeasures for biological weapons, antimicrobials targeting ultraresistant bacteria, and treatments for infectious diseases with pandemic potential. The commercial upside for these therapies is inherently limited because they are developed with the understanding that they should only be used in exceptional cases. In addition, widespread use of antimicrobials for ultraresistant infections would lead to resistance to these treatments, undermining their usefulness. Therefore, as Box 4-4 describes, there are few market incentives to develop these critically important therapies because of their limited use profiles.

Length and Cost of Clinical Trial

The duration, and therefore the cost, of clinical trials can also affect investment decisions in certain therapeutic areas. Recruitment into clinical trials can be more challenging, and therefore more expensive, for some

BOX 4-4
Understanding Barriers to Antimicrobial Drug Development

According to the National Institutes of Health, antibiotic-resistant bacterial infections cause more than a million deaths globally each year, a number predicted to increase without the development of new, targeted antibiotics (NIH, 2024a). In the face of a dire need for innovation in antimicrobial (AM) drug development, a 2023 World Health Organization review of clinical and preclinical development in this area identified "a glaring insufficiency in novel approaches in the R&D pipeline to effectively combat the increasing emergence and spread of antimicrobial resistance" (Global AMR R&D Hub and WHO, 2023; Third World Network Berhad, 2024).

The lack of research and innovation around AM drugs is well known and is evidenced by a consensus in the literature (NASEM, 2017; Renwick and Mossialos, 2018; Sertkaya et al., 2022). Despite this, a dearth of research and development into these drugs continues, largely because of market forces that prevent investment into such drug development. A 2022 Department of Health and Human Services report notes that the most significant challenge for drug developers is that returns for AM drugs are significantly lower than for other pharmaceuticals (Sertkaya et al., 2022). A 2017 economic analysis estimated the cost of developing an AM drug at about $1.5 billion (Towse et al., 2017). However, the same analysis showed the anticipated revenue from sales of an AM is about $46 million per year.

The purpose of new AM drugs is to address drug-resistant bacteria, as a wide range of AM drugs to treat most bacteria already exist. Therefore, because these new AM drugs would be used sparingly to limit the emergence of further AM-resistant bacteria, the market for new AM drugs is relatively small. Furthermore, because a single course of treatment for AM drugs is short, as is the corresponding revenue, there is little profit to be made from these medications. Many countries' government agencies play a role in setting drug prices (see Chapter 5), so manufacturers are not able to set high prices for new AM drugs, especially when compared to other AM drugs, which are very low in cost. AM drugs do not cost more than a few thousands of dollars for a course of treatment, as compared with cancer drugs, which can cost over $100,000 per year (Blaskovich et al., 2017; Sertkaya et al., 2022). The continuous shift in the types of AM resistance in bacterial pathogens creates further challenges for drug developers since by the time an AM drug makes it to market, there may be significantly less demand for it, with the emergence of newer strains of resistant organisms (Sertkaya et al., 2022). For example, the

continued

BOX 4-4 Continued

pharmaceutical company Achaogen, which successfully developed a Food and Drug Administration–approved antibiotic to treat drug-resistant infections, filed for Chapter 11 bankruptcy in 2019 (Blewett et al., 2019). Even with a successful product, the company was unable to have commercial success.

Therefore, despite the consensus on the need for more drug development in this space, it is unlikely that without intervention, which could take various forms, these necessary treatments will be developed. As Blaskovich et al. (2017) state:

> We are facing a potential catastrophe of untreatable bacterial infections, driven by the inexorable rise of extensively drug-resistant bacteria, coupled with a market failure of pharmaceutical and biotech companies to deliver new therapeutic options. While global recognition of the problem is finally apparent, solutions are still a long way from being implemented. (p. 103)

---

diseases. For example, many trials for mental health conditions, such as depression, are particularly challenging for recruitment. For example, one study offering cognitive behavioral therapy by computer had enrollment rates ranging from 2 percent to 60 percent and actual participation rates of 3 percent to 25 percent (Kaltenthaler et al., 2008). In another study examining treating diabetes in individuals with depression, recruitment into the study took over double the amount of time initially budgeted (Myers et al., 2019). This likely influences investment decisions, perhaps decreasing potential investment into these more difficult-to-recruit diseases and conditions.

The length of the trials is also one of the reasons that there is a lack of investment in preventative therapeutics or early-stage interventions. For example, an early-stage intervention for preventing cancer can take decades to observe outcomes (e.g., the development of cancer), depending on the natural history of a particular tumor type, and speed of progression (Serrano et al., 2019). The length of these trials and the amount of follow-up required to show evidence of efficacy is cost-prohibitive for many companies. Therefore, cancer innovation tends to focus on later-stage cancer therapies, where trials can be run more quickly and for lower cost as the prognosis for patients with late-stage cancer is often poor and survival is a key endpoint for many of these trials (Budish et al., 2015). One potential solution to these lengthy clinical trials is to expeditiously develop and validate surrogate endpoints. Although these endpoints are not direct measures of clinical benefit, if they are reasonable predictors of clinical benefit, they can be used to more rapidly evaluate efficacy (FDA, 2019). With the development and use of better surrogate endpoints for early-stage cancer therapies, patients could get access to medications that are reasonably expected to have an effect, with the expectation that manufacturers will confirm clinical benefit at a later date.

Scientifically Complex Populations

There are certain populations that are scientifically complex, such as pregnant or lactating individuals and pediatric populations, making research in these populations more costly and therefore less likely to occur. Although there are unique challenges for each population, there is a mismatch in investment in innovations compared with the disease burdens that affect each group.

Pediatric drug development has lagged behind research to address adult conditions. In addition to heightened ethical scrutiny, pediatric clinical trials require specialized expertise to properly evaluate pharmacokinetics, pharmacodynamics, and efficacy in children as they age (IOM, 2012). Furthermore, recruitment for pediatric trials often requires more trial sites than adult trials to recruit sufficient numbers of participants across age groups. Most pediatric conditions are also considered rare, which presents some of the same challenges outlined in the earlier section about small patient populations (Speer et al., 2023). Congress has passed legislation creating financial incentives and regulatory requirements to encourage research for pediatric populations (see Chapter 5 for more details), and these have been helpful in getting more pediatric information in drug labeling (FDA, 2022). However, most drugs used in children still do not contain pediatric prescribing information, and this continues to be the case, even for new drugs with a postmarketing requirement to conduct pediatric studies (Carmack et al., 2020).

Pregnant and lactating populations are also scientifically complex and, similar to pediatric populations, require additional resources to conduct research (NASEM, 2024a). Although ethical considerations and liability concerns are often raised as barriers to conducting research with these populations, evidence supports the ethical case for including these populations in research (NASEM, 2024a; Task Force on Research Specific to Pregnant Women and Lactating Women, 2018; WHO, 2023), and there is little evidence of increased liability for clinical trials involving pregnant or lactating populations (NASEM, 2024a). However, given the increased cost associated with conducting research with these populations and given that pregnant and lactating women can be prescribed medications without specific labeling information, there is little financial incentive to conduct research with these populations (NASEM, 2024a). This lack of incentives prevents innovation and investment for research on high-burden diseases with large unmet needs that affect these populations, such as preeclampsia, preterm birth, gestational diabetes, and hyperemesis gravidarum.

All of the market forces covered in this section contribute to continued unmet needs for diseases and conditions that have high disease burdens. These market forces contribute to the misalignment discussed in Chapter 3. The next chapter reviews the levers that policy makers can use—and have used—to address some of the factors discussed in this section and ultimately reduce the misalignment in investments for diseases with high burdens and unmet needs.

Finding 4-2: Despite early signs of efficacy or even FDA approval of a drug, some therapeutics are shelved or pulled from the market because there is not a large enough economic incentive or return on investment for a company to fully develop the drug or continue manufacturing it once approved.

REFERENCES

Abi-Dargham, A., S. J. Moeller, F. Ali, C. Delorenzo, K. Domschke, G. Horga, A. Jutla, R. Kotov, M. P. Paulus, J. M. Rubio, G. Sanacora, J. Veenstra-Vanderweele, and J. H. Krystal. 2023. Candidate biomarkers in psychiatric disorders: State of the field. *World Psychiatry* 22(2):236–262.

Acemoglu, D., and J. Linn. 2004. Market size in innovation: Theory and evidence from the pharmaceutical industry. *Quarterly Journal of Economics* 119(3):1049–1090.

Ackley, S. F., S. C. Zimmerman, W. D. Brenowitz, E. J. Tchetgen Tchetgen, A. L. Gold, J. J. Manly, E. R. Mayeda, T. J. Filshtein, M. C. Power, F. M. Elahi, A. M. Brickman, and M. M. Glymour. 2021. Effect of reductions in amyloid levels on cognitive change in randomized trials: Instrumental variable meta-analysis. *BMJ* 372:156.

Alzheimer's Association. 2024. *Alzheimer's disease facts and figures.* https://www.alz.org/alzheimers-dementia/facts-figures (accessed April 14, 2025).

Alzheimer's Association. n.d. *Research funding.* https://www.alz.org/get-involved-now/advocate/research-funding (accessed March 17, 2025).

American Lung Association. 2024a. *COPD in your state.* https://www.lung.org/lung-health-diseases/lung-disease-lookup/copd/for-health-professionals/copd-in-your-state (accessed March 3, 2025).

American Lung Association. 2024b. *Diagnosing COPD.* https://www.lung.org/lung-health-diseases/lung-disease-lookup/copd/symptoms-diagnosis/diagnosing (accessed April 14, 2025).

Ashton, N. J., W. S. Brum, G. Di Molfetta, A. L. Benedet, B. Arslan, E. Jonaitis, R. E. Langhough, K. Cody, R. Wilson, C. M. Carlsson, E. Vanmechelen, L. Montoliu-Gaya, J. Lantero-Rodriguez, N. Rahmouni, C. Tissot, J. Stevenson, S. Servaes, J. Therriault, T. Pascoal, A. Lleó, D. Alcolea, J. Fortea, P. Rosa-Neto, S. Johnson, A. Jeromin, K. Blennow, and H. Zetterberg. 2024. Diagnostic accuracy of a plasma phosphorylated tau 217 immunoassay for Alzheimer disease pathology. *JAMA Neurology* 81(3):255–263.

ASPE (Assistant Secretary for Planning and Evaluation). 2024. Comparing U.S. and international market size and average pricing for prescription drugs, 2017-2022. https:// aspe.hhs.gov/sites/default/files/documents/4326cc7fe43bc11770598cf2a13f478c/ international-market-size-prices.pdf (accessed April 21, 2025).

Barnes, P. J., S. Bonini, W. Seeger, M. G. Belvisi, B. Ward, and A. Holmes. 2015. Barriers to new drug development in respiratory disease. *European Respiratory Journal* 45(5):1197–1207.

Begley, S. 2019. The maddening saga of how an Alzheimer's "cabal" thwarted progress toward a cure for decades. *STAT News*, June 25. https://www.statnews.com/2019/06/25/ alzheimers-cabal-thwarted-progress-toward-cure/ (accessed March 17, 2025).

Blaskovich, M. A., M. S. Butler, and M. A. Cooper. 2017. Polishing the tarnished silver bullet: The quest for new antibiotics. *Essays in Biochemistry* 61(1):103–114.

Blewett, M., B. Kocher, and B. Shady. 2019. How to cure the antibiotic industry's profitability infection. *Fortune.* https://fortune.com/2019/11/14/antibiotics-funding-achaogen-tetraphase-pharmaceuticals/ (accessed May 15, 2025).

Blume-Kohout, M. E., and N. Sood. 2013. Market size and innovation: Effects of Medicare Part D on pharmaceutical research and development. *Journal of Public Economics* 97:327–336.

Budish, E., B. N. Roin, and H. Williams. 2015. Do firms underinvest in long-term research? Evidence from cancer clinical trials. *American Economic Review* 105(7):2044–2085.

Bureau of Economic Analysis. 2018. *Durable goods.* https://www.bea.gov/help/glossary/ durable-goods (accessed April 21, 2025).

Carmack, M., T. Hwang, and F. T. Bourgeois. 2020. Pediatric drug policies supporting safe and effective use of therapeutics in children: A systematic analysis. *Health Affairs (Millwood)* 39(10):1799–1805.

Cohen, J. P. 2024. New non-opioid pain meds hold promise, but face clinical development and insurer challenges. *Forbes.* https://www.forbes.com/sites/joshuacohen/2024/03/18/ new-non-opioid-pain-meds-hold-promise-but-face-clinical-development-and-insurer-challenges/ (accessed April 14, 2025).

Cohen, B., L. J. Ruth, and C. V. Preuss. 2025. Opioid analgesics. In *StatPearls*. Treasure Island, FL: StatPearls Publishing. https://www.ncbi.nlm.nih.gov/books/NBK459161/ (accessed May 30, 2025).

Congressional Budget Office. 2021. *Research and development in the pharmaceutical industry.* https://www.cbo.gov/publication/57126#_idTextAnchor036 (accessed April 14, 2025).

Cubanski, J. 2024. A current snapshot of the Medicare Part D prescription drug benefit. *KFF*, October 9. https://www.kff.org/medicare/issue-brief/a-current-snapshot-of-the-medicare-part-d-prescription-drug-benefit/#:~:text=Part%20D%20plans%20are%20 required,anticonvulsants%2C%20antiretrovirals%2C%20and%20antineoplastics (accessed April 21, 2025).

Cubanski, J., M. Rae, K. Young, and A. Damico. 2019. How does prescription drug spending and use compare across large employer plans, Medicare Part D, and Medicaid? *KFF*, May 20. https://www.kff.org/medicare/issue-brief/how-does-prescription-drug-spending-and-use-compare-across-large-employer-plans-medicare-part-d-and-medicaid/ (accessed January 2, 2025).

Cummings, J. L., D. P. Goldman, N. R. Simmons-Stern, and E. Ponton. 2022. The costs of developing treatments for Alzheimer's disease: A retrospective exploration. *Alzheimer's & Dementia* 18(3):469–477.

Dansie, E. J., and D. C. Turk. 2013. Assessment of patients with chronic pain. *British Journal of Anaesthesia* 111(1):19–25.

Davey, S., K. Costello, M. Russo, S. Davies, H. S. Lalani, A. S. Kesselheim, and B. N. Rome. 2024. Changes in use of hepatitis C direct-acting antivirals after access restrictions were eased by state Medicaid programs. *JAMA Health Forum* 5(4):e240302.

Derry, S., P. Conaghan, J. A. Da Silva, P. J. Wiffen, and R. A. Moore. 2016. Topical NSAIDS for chronic musculoskeletal pain in adults. *Cochrane Database Systematic Reviews* 4(4):Cd007400.

Dickson, S., N. Gabriel, and I. Hernandez. 2023. Changes in net prices and spending for pharmaceuticals after the introduction of new therapeutic competition, 2011–19. *Health Affairs* 42(8):1062–1070.

Dolan, R. 2019. Understanding the Medicaid prescription drug rebate program. *KFF*, April 25. https://www.kff.org/medicaid/issue-brief/understanding-the-medicaid-prescription-drug-rebate-program/ (accessed April 21, 2025).

Dolan, R., R. Garfield, and R. Rudowitz. 2021. Potential implications of policy changes in Medicaid drug purchasing. *KFF*, May 4. https://www.kff.org/report-section/potential-implications-of-policy-changes-in-medicaid-drug-purchasing-issue-brief/ (accessed May 21, 2025).

Dowell, D., T. M. Haegerich, and R. Chou. 2016. CDC guideline for prescribing opioids for chronic pain—United States, 2016. *JAMA* 315(15):1624–1645.

Eisenberg, R. S. 2019. Opting into device regulation in the face of uncertain patentability. *Marquette Intellectual Property Law Review* 23(1):1–19.

Favretti, M., C. Iannuccelli, and M. Di Franco. 2023. Pain biomarkers in fibromyalgia syndrome: Current understanding and future directions. *International Journal of Molecular Science* 24(13):10443.

FDA (Food and Drug Administration). 2014. *In vitro companion diagnostic devices: Guidance for industry and Food and Drug Administration staff.* Center for Devices and Radiological Health, Center for Biologics Evaluation and Research, and Center for Drug Evaluation and Research. https://www.fda.gov/media/81309/download (accessed April 14, 2025).

FDA. 2019. *Demonstrating substantial evidence of effectiveness for human drug and biological products.* Draft guidance for industry. Docket no. FDA-2019-D-4964. https://www.fda.gov/regulatory-information/search-fda-guidance-documents/demonstrating-substantial-evidence-effectiveness-human-drug-and-biological-products (accessed April 22, 2025).

FDA. 2022. Historic milestone: 1,000 drugs, biologics have new pediatric use information in labeling. *AAP News*, September 1. https://www.fda.gov/media/161414/download?attachment, 2022 (accessed March 14, 2025).

FDA. 2023. *Highlights of prescribing information: Leqembi.* https://www.accessdata.fda.gov/Drugsatfda_docs/Label/2023/761269Orig1s001lbl.Pdf (accessed April 14, 2025).

FDA. 2024a. *Highlights of prescribing information: Kisunla.* https://www.fda.gov/media/180803/download (accessed April 14, 2025).

FDA. 2024b. *Rare diseases at the FDA.* https://www.fda.gov/patients/rare-diseases-fda (accessed March 20, 2025).

FDA. 2025. *FDA clears first blood test used in diagnosing Alzheimer's disease.* https://www.fda.gov/news-events/press-announcements/fda-clears-first-blood-test-used-used-diagnosing-alzheimers-disease (accessed May 21, 2025).

Fleurence, R. L., and F. S. Collins. 2023. A national hepatitis C elimination program in the United States. *JAMA* 329(15):1251.

Fonseca, D. A., I. Amaral, A. C. Pinto, and M. D. Cotrim. 2019. Orphan drugs: Major development challenges at the clinical stage. *Drug Discovery Today* 24(3):867–872.

Gallo, A. 2014. A refresher on net present value. *Harvard Business Review*, https://hbr.org/2014/11/a-refresher-on-net-present-value (accessed April 11, 2025).

Global AMR R&D Hub and WHO (World Health Organization). 2023. *Incentivising the development of new antibacterial treatments 2023.* Geneva, Switzerland: Global AMR R&D Hub and WHO.

Goldman, D., and D. Lakdawalla. 2018. *The global burden of medical innovation.* https://schaeffer.usc.edu/wp-content/uploads/2024/10/01.2018_Global20Burden20of20Medical20Innovation.pdf (accessed May 30, 2025).

Green Park Collaborative. 2015. *Initial medical policy and model coverage guidelines for clinical next generation sequencing in oncology: Report and recommendations.* Baltimore, MD: Center for Medical Technology Policy. https://www.cmtpnet.org/docs/resources/ Full_Release_Version_August_13__2015.pdf (accessed April 14, 2025).

Greenleaf, E. A., E. J. Johnson, V. G. Morwitz, and E. Shalev. 2016. The price does not include additional taxes, fees, and surcharges: A review of research on partitioned pricing. *Journal of Consumer Psychology* 26(1):105–124.

Haendel, M., N. Vasilevsky, D. Unni, C. Bologa, N. Harris, H. Rehm, A. Hamosh, G. Baynam, T. Groza, J. McMurry, H. Dawkins, A. Rath, C. Thaxton, G. Bocci, M. P. Joachimiak, S. Köhler, P. N. Robinson, C. Mungall, and T. I. Oprea. 2020. How many rare diseases are there? *Nature Reviews Drug Discovery* 19(2):77–78.

Hernandez, I., and A. Hung. 2024. A primer on brand-name prescription drug reimbursement in the United States. *Journal of Managed Care & Specialty Pharmacy* 30(1):99–106.

Hwang, T. J., X. Qin, N. L. Keating, H. A. Huskamp, and S. B. Dusetzina. 2022. Assessment of out-of-pocket costs with rebate pass-through for brand-name cancer drugs under Medicare Part D. *JAMA Oncology* 8(1):155–156.

ICER (Institute for Clinical and Economic Review). 2023. *Lecanemab for early Alzheimer's disease.* https://icer.org/wp-content/uploads/2023/04/ICER_Alzheimers-Disease_Final-Report_For-Publication_04172023.pdf (accessed April 14, 2025).

IOM (Institute of Medicine). 2012. *Safe and effective medicines for children: Pediatric studies conducted under the Best Pharmaceuticals for Children Act and the Pediatric Research Equity Act.* Washington, DC: The National Academies Press.

Kaltenthaler, E., P. Sutcliffe, G. Parry, C. Beverley, A. Rees, and M. Ferriter. 2008. The acceptability to patients of computerized cognitive behaviour therapy for depression: A systematic review. *Psychological Medicine* 38(11):1521–1530.

Kaushik, A. C., A. Kumar, Z. Peng, A. Khan, M. Junaid, A. Ali, S. Bharadwaj, and D.-Q. Wei. 2019. Evaluation and validation of synergistic effects of amyloid-beta inhibitor–gold nanoparticles complex on Alzheimer's disease using deep neural network approach. *Journal of Materials Research* 34(11):1845–1853.

Kempf, L., J. C. Goldsmith, and R. Temple. 2018. Challenges of developing and conducting clinical trials in rare disorders. *American Journal of Medical Genetics Part A* 176(4):773–783.

Kingwell, K. 2025. FDA approves new non-opioid pain drug. *Nature Reviews Drug Discovery* 24(3):158.

Kirby, K. N. 1997. Bidding on the future: Evidence against normative discounting of delayed rewards. *Journal of Experimental Psychology: General* 126(1):54–70.

Klomp, C. 2025. *Draft guidance on the Medicare Drug Price Negotiation Program.* Centers for Medicare & Medicaid Services, May 12. https://www.cms.gov/files/document/ipay-2028-draft-guidance.pdf (accessed May 16, 2025).

Kochanek, K. D., S. L. Murphy, J. Xu, and E. Arias. *National Center for Health Statistics. 2022. Data brief 492. Mortality in the Uunited States, 2022.* https://www.cdc.gov/nchs/ products/databriefs/db492.htm (accessed April 14, 2025).

Krishnamurthy, N., A. A. Grimshaw, S. A. Axson, S. H. Choe, and J. E. Miller. 2022. Drug repurposing: A systematic review on root causes, barriers and facilitators. *BMC Health Services Research* 22(1).

Lee, K., J. Choi, and Y. J. Li. 2014. Regulatory focus as a predictor of attitudes toward partitioned and combined pricing. *Journal of Consumer Psychology* 24(3):355–362.

Leung, J. M., M. E. Obeidat, M. Sadatsafavi, and D. D. Sin. 2019. Introduction to precision medicine in COPD. *European Respiratory Journal* 53(4):1802460.

Levis, B., A. Benedetti, and B. D. Thombs. 2019. Accuracy of patient health questionnaire-9 (PHQ-9) for screening to detect major depression: Individual participant data meta-analysis. *BMJ* 365:l1476.

Morwitz, V. G., E. A. Greenleaf, and E. J. Johnson. 1998. Divide and prosper: Consumers' reactions to partitioned prices. *Journal of Marketing Research* 35(4):453–463.

Myers, B. A., Y. Pillay, W. Guyton Hornsby, J. Shubrook, C. Saha, K. J. Mather, K. Fitzpatrick, and M. de Groot. 2019. Recruitment effort and costs from a multi-center randomized controlled trial for treating depression in type 2 diabetes. *Trials* 20(1):621.

NASEM (National Academies of Sciences, Engineering, and Medicine). 2017. *Combating antimicrobial resistance: A One Health approach to a global threat: Proceedings of a workshop*. Washington, DC: The National Academies Press.

NASEM. 2018. *Advancing therapeutic development for pain and opioid use disorders through public-private partnerships: Proceedings of a workshop*. Edited by L. Bain, S. M. P. Norris, and C. Stroud. Washington, DC: The National Academies Press.

NASEM. 2024a. *Advancing clinical research with pregnant and lactating populations: Overcoming real and perceived liability risks*. Washington, DC: The National Academies Press.

NASEM. 2024b. *Regulatory processes for rare disease drugs in the United States and European Union: Flexibilities and collaborative opportunities*. Washington, DC: The National Academies Press.

Niazi, S. K. 2024. The United States Food and Drug Administration's platform technology designation to expedite the development of drugs. *Pharmaceutics* 16(7):918.

NIH (National Institutes of Health). 2024a. *NIH research matters: Designing a new antibiotic to combat drug resistance*. https://www.nih.gov/news-events/nih-research-matters/designing-new-antibiotic-combat-drug-resistance (accessed April 15, 2025).

NIH. 2024b. *The helping to end addiction long-term® initiative*. https://heal.nih.gov/ (accessed April 14, 2025).

Paladini, A., J. Barrientos Penaloza, R. Plancarte Sanchez, T. Ergönenç, and G. Varrassi. 2023. Bridging old and new in pain medicine: An historical review. *Cureus* 15(8):e43639.

Pang, M., L. Zhu, A. Gabelle, A. R. Gafson, R. W. Platt, J. E. Galvin, P. Krolak-Salmon, I. Rubino, C. de Moor, S. Belachew, and C. Shen. 2023. Effect of reduction in brain amyloid levels on change in cognitive and functional decline in randomized clinical trials: An instrumental variable meta-analysis. *Alzheimer's & Dementia* 19(4):1292–1299.

Paul, D., G. Sanap, S. Shenoy, D. Kalyane, K. Kalia, and R. K. Tekade. 2021. Artificial intelligence in drug discovery and development. *Drug Discovery Today* 26(1):80–93.

Pauly, M. V. 2017. The questionable economic case for value-based drug pricing in market health systems. *Value Health* 20(2):278–282.

Piller, C. 2022. Scientists tie third clinical trial death to experimental Alzheimer's drug. *Science*, December 21. https://www.science.org/content/article/scientists-tie-third-clinical-trial-death-experimental-alzheimer-s-drug (accessed March 20, 2025).

Renwick, M., and E. Mossialos. 2018. What are the economic barriers of antibiotic R&D and how can we overcome them? *Expert Opinion on Drug Discovery* 13(10):889–892.

Rikard, S. M., A. E. Strahan, K. M. Schmit, and P. Guy Jr. 2023. Chronic pain among adults—United States, 2019–2021. *MMWR Morbidity Mortality Weekly Report* 72:379–385. http://dx.doi.org/10.15585/mmwr.mm7215a1.

Robinson-Papp, J., M. C. George, D. Dorfman, and D. M. Simpson. 2015. Barriers to chronic pain measurement: A qualitative study of patient perspectives. *Pain Medicine* 16(7):1256–1264.

Selkoe, D. J. 2025. There is no "amyloid cabal" in Alzheimer's research. *STAT News*, February 14. https://www.statnews.com/2025/02/14/alzheimers-doctored-charles-piller-amyloid-hypothesis/ (accessed March 17, 2025).

Serrano, D., B. Bonanni, and K. Brown. 2019. Therapeutic cancer prevention: Achievements and ongoing challenges—A focus on breast and colorectal cancer. *Molecular Oncology* 13(3):579–590.

Sertkaya, A., A. Berlind, J. D. McGeeney, C. Berger, and O. Stokes-Cawley. 2022. Analysis of market challenges for antimicrobial drug development in the United States: Final report [internet]. Washington, DC: Office of the Assistant Secretary for Planning and Evaluation. https://www.ncbi.nlm.nih.gov/books/NBK602559/pdf/Bookshelf_NBK602559.pdf (accessed April 14, 2025).

Sertkaya, A., T. Beleche, A. Jessup, and B. D. Sommers. 2024. Costs of drug development and research and development intensity in the U.S., 2000–2018. *JAMA Network Open* 7(6):e2415445.

Speer, E. M., L. K. Lee, F. T. Bourgeois, D. Gitterman, W. W. Hay, J. M. Davis, and J. R. Javier. 2023. The state and future of pediatric research—An introductory overview. *Pediatric Research*. https://doi.org/10.1038/s41390-022-02439-4.

Staudt, M. D. 2022. The multidisciplinary team in pain management. *Neurosurgery Clinics of North America* 33(3):241–249.

Task Force on Research Specific to Pregnant Women and Lactating Women. 2018. *Report to Secretary, Health and Human Services and Congress.* https://www.nichd.nih.gov/sites/default/files/2018-09/PRGLAC_Report.pdf (accessed April 14, 2025).

Tax Policy Center Urban Institute & Brookings Institution. n.d. What are state balanced budget requirements and how do they work? In *The Tax Policy Briefing Book.* Urban Institute & Brookings Institution. https://taxpolicycenter.org/news/unrigging-economy-will-require-enforcing-tax-laws (accessed April 21, 2025).

Towse, A., C. K. Hoyle, J. Goodall, M. Hirsch, J. Mestre-Ferrandiz, and J. H. Rex. 2017. Time for a change in how new antibiotics are reimbursed: Development of an insurance framework for funding new antibiotics based on a policy of risk mitigation. *Health Policy* 121(10):1025–1030.

Third World Network Berhad. 2024. *Health: Not enough "trail-blazing" drugs to fight deadly bacteria, warns WHO.* TWN: Third World Network Berhad. https://twn.my/title2/health.info/2024/hi240603.htm (accessed April 21, 2025).

Vavassori, S., S. Russell, C. Scotti, and S. Benvenuti. 2024. Unlocking the full potential of rare disease drug development: Exploring the not-for-profit sector's contributions to drug development and access. *Frontiers in Pharmacology* 15:1441807.

Waldron, J. 2023. 'We're swimming against the tide': Why Lilly is trying new strokes to persevere against pain. *Fierce Biotech.* https://www.fiercebiotech.com/biotech/were-swimming-against-tide-why-lilly-trying-new-strokes-persevere-against-pain (accessed April 14, 2025).

Walsh, S., R. Merrick, E. Richard, S. Nurock, and C. Brayne. 2022. Lecanemab for Alzheimer's disease. *BMJ* 379:o3010.

Werble, C. 2017. Formularies. *Health Affairs.* In *Presciption drug pricing: A Health Affairs collection.* Bethesda, MD: Health Affairs. https://www.healthaffairs.org/pb-assets/documents/collected-works/collected-works-prescription-drug-pricing-1525875761187.pdf?download (accessed April 14, 2025).

WHO (World Health Organization). 2023. *Supplementary report on implementing WHA resolution 75.8 on strengthening clinical trials to provide high-quality evidence on health interventions and to improve research quality and coordination.* Geneva, Switzerland: World Health Organization.

Wouters, O. J., and A. S. Kesselheim. 2024. Quantifying research and development expenditures in the drug industry. *JAMA Network Open* 7(6):e2415407.

Xue, Q. C., and L. L. Ouellette. 2020. Innovation policy and the market for vaccines. *Journal of Law and the Biosciences* 7(1):lsaa026.

Yates, N., and J. Hinkel. 2022. The economics of moonshots: Value in rare disease drug development. *Clinical Translational Science* 15(4):809–812.

Zhang, W., Y. Li, W. Ren, and B. Liu. 2023. Artificial intelligence technology in Alzheimer's disease research. *Intractable & Rare Diseases Research* 12(4):208–212.

Zissimopoulos, J., E. Crimmins, and P. St Clair. 2014. The value of delaying Alzheimer's disease onset. *Forum for Health Economics Policy* 18(1):25–39.

5

Strategies to Better Align Innovations with Disease Burden and Unmet Need

The government has a number of existing policies and programs to encourage innovation in drug development, including several focused specifically on addressing unmet need. Among them are National Institutes of Health (NIH) and other government funding for science; certain Food and Drug Administration (FDA) policies and programs to promote investment, support scientific advancement, and speed drugs to market; and incentives established by Congress, such as those relating to rare and pediatric disease research and development. Various aspects of government funded (and private-market) drug coverage and reimbursement also create incentives and disincentives for drug development. Figure 5-1 provides an overview of the actors that can improve alignment between investment and unmet needs along the drug development cycle, as well as the different levers that can be used to drive changes by these actors. Although this figure depicts the cycle as linear, it is really a cycle that feeds back on itself. This chapter will discuss each of these levers for change in detail.

NIH AND PUBLIC FUNDING

As discussed in Chapter 3, NIH is a key player in the funding of innovative therapeutics through its support of research in basic science, disease biology, and epidemiology. This has contributed significantly to the development of new drugs and provides the foundation by which industry studies advance and serve to derisk investment in new technologies. Publicly funded research has been said to be the "foundation upon which complementary

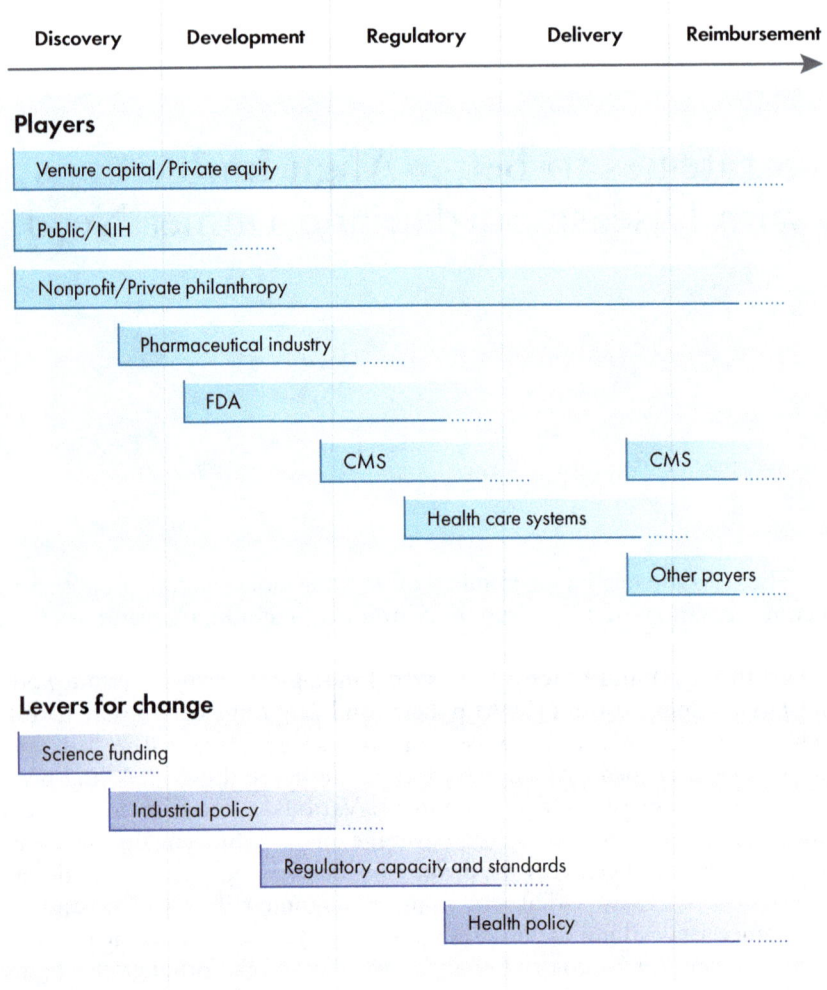

FIGURE 5-1 Framework of the drug development cycle, mapped with players and levers for change.

work on the applied science of drug development could be undertaken by the private sector" (Congressional Budget Office, 2021).

With NIH providing the bulk of funding for basic research, studies indicate that industry investment costs in new drug approvals were cut by nearly half, creating economic efficiencies that make it possible for numerous companies to develop individual products (Galkina Cleary et al., 2023). These and other data indicate that NIH and other public funding is crucial in pharmaceutical discovery (Ledley and Galkina Cleary, 2023).

In addition to funding most early-stage biomedical research in the United States, NIH also funds some later-stage development, including translational research and clinical trials. These efforts occur through both its disease-focused institutes (often coordinating with the NIH Clinical Center) and its separate translation-focused programs—the National Center for Advancing Translational Sciences (NCATS) and the Advanced Research Projects Agency for Health (ARPA-H), discussed later in this section. NIH also directly funds commercialization efforts by providing nondilutive funding to small business to develop early-stage technologies through the Small Business Innovation Research (SBIR) program and the Small Business Technology Transfer (STTR) program. More details on the SBIR/STTR programs can be found below.

While it is clear that NIH-funded research is critical to advancing innovation, NIH processes do not clearly prioritize funding for disease areas with high disease burdens and unmet needs. To better understand why, it is helpful to understand the process for setting funding priorities within NIH.

NIH Funding Process

Rather than funding NIH broadly and allowing NIH leadership to allocate funds between each of 27 NIH institutes and centers (ICs), Congress appropriates funds for the ICs directly; those congressional funds broadly determine the amount of money that each IC can distribute. This process begins from the bottom up, with each IC discussing priorities with the NIH director. The NIH director then negotiates the budget for each institute and center with the Department of Health and Human Services (HHS) and the Office of Management and Budget (OMB) but is not able to communicate directly with Congress on funding priorities (IOM, 1998). Congress then appropriates funds to each IC at NIH, taking into account the budget and priorities of the administration. However, Congress does not explicitly consider disease burden or unmet need when allocating funding for each IC (Pierson and Millum, 2022), and, as discussed earlier, Congress does not necessarily have the requisite data to allow for such decision making.

Each IC then determines how to allocate its funds, incorporating input from a number of sources. Each IC has its own mission, budget, leadership, and funding strategies. However, a significant amount of funding goes toward collaborative funding across ICs, such as activities on women's health, pain, brain health, chronic diseases, pediatric studies, and others. Funding decisions are made taking into account a number of factors, such as scientific merit, scientific opportunity, current portfolio, congressional mandates (for research on specific diseases, beyond their appropriations for individual institutes and centers), and public health needs. Although disease burden and unmet needs could be considered in a number of these categories, they are not explicitly considered when ICs set their funding priorities.

Each IC has a strategic plan, a director, and advisory councils that help determine the topics for solicited research, such as program announcements, notices of special interest, or requests for information. To decide which research project grants get funded through these solicitations, NIH uses a two-step process for review. First is a peer-review process, using the recently updated Simplified Review Framework, followed by review by the IC advisory council. The new simplified framework for NIH scoring criteria takes three main factors into account for each research project grant: (1) importance of the research; (2) rigor and feasibility; and (3) expertise and resources. Considerations about disease burden and unmet needs could be considered in the importance of research score. However, they are not explicitly addressed as a factor to be examined when scoring the importance of research section. By including considerations of disease burden and unmet need in this scoring criteria, investigators would at least be incentivized to consider how the research they are undertaking meets these important criteria.

As noted in prior chapters, one key barrier to addressing unmet need is gaps in scientific knowledge. The knowledge gaps are best filled through robust government funding into basic science and disease epidemiology, which can elucidate new and promising pathways for drug development. Despite this need for innovative and novel work, NIH has long faced criticisms that it does not fund enough innovative, high-risk/high-reward ideas. For example, grants that include substantial preliminary data and investigators with substantial prior NIH funding and experience are more likely to be funded than new ideas and investigators. In complex areas of science, this can reduce opportunities for novel approaches. For example, NIH has been criticized by its focus on amyloid-targeting therapies for treating Alzheimer's disease at the expense of other potentially promising avenues, although what is considered a promising avenue may be rather subjective (Piller, 2022).

According to a paper published for the Building a Better NIH project (Sampat et al., 2023), the two strategies to resolve this challenge are to change the peer-review system for evaluating grants or to create programs that specifically target funding for research with a high risk of failure but also a high probability of innovative effect if successful. Although the new review criteria may help with some of this, particularly by reducing reputational bias that previously favored more senior, established investigators, truly new ideas may not have enough "preliminary data" or be "derisked" enough to obtain funding (NIH, 2024b). Therefore, it is important for NIH to explore creating new programs that specifically fund risky research, especially ones that explicitly target unmet needs. Although NIH does currently have a program through the Common Fund for high-risk, high-reward research (Box 5-1), this program does not explicitly take disease burden and unmet needs into account.

BOX 5-1
NIH High-Risk, High Reward Research

The National Institutes of Health (NIH) currently has funding opportunities for innovative and novel research ideas through the NIH Common Fund. The NIH Common Fund refers to funds allocated through the Office of the Director to support "bold scientific programs that catalyze discovery across all biomedical and behavioral research" (NIH Common Fund, 2025).

One of the programs funded through the Common Fund is the High-Risk, High-Reward research program, which aims to support highly innovative research with the potential for broad impact within the NIH mission. According to the website, this program consists of four NIH director's awards to support this effort, with stated efforts as follows:

1. The NIH Director's Pioneer Award funds scientists with outstanding records of creativity pursuing pioneering approaches to major challenges.
2. The NIH Director's New Innovator Award awards exceptionally creative early-career scientists proposing innovative, high-impact projects.
3. The NIH Director's Transformative Research Award is for individuals or teams proposing groundbreaking, unconventional research with the potential to create new scientific paradigms.
4. The NIH Director's Early Independence Award funds exceptional junior scientists bypassing postdoctoral training to launch independent research careers.

In 2024, the High-Risk, High-Reward program awarded 67 awards totaling over $207 million (about 0.4 percent of the NIH budget) to investigators to fund their research projects (NIH, 2024a).

SBIR/STTR Grant Programs

SBIR/STTR grants, collectively known as America's Seed Fund, provide nondilutive funding to American small businesses for the development and commercialization of innovative technologies (SEED, n.d.). Nondilutive funding is advantageous for early-stage companies because it provides capital without requiring companies to give up equity, and thus aligns financial incentives for teams involved in innovation. Key components of the federal SBIR/STTR support include the Small Business Administration (SBA), which coordinates America's Seed Fund across 12 participating federal agencies; support organizations, such as accelerators and technical assistance centers that support applicants; federal agencies that fund qualified proposals; and entrepreneurs who apply for awards and collaborate with agencies to develop their technologies (SBA, 2025). Funding phases for the SBIR/STTR programs include:

- Phase I: Initial funding to explore the technical merit or feasibility of an idea or technology
- Phase II: Continuation of research and development (R&D) efforts initiated in phase I, moving toward prototype development
- Phase III: Commercialization stage, where private-sector funding or non-SBIR/STTR federal funding supports the final development and market entry

The program is intended to bridge academia and industry and thereby promote technology transfer and address translational challenges that small companies face when commercializing new discoveries. In addition, SBIR/STTR grants help derisk early-stage technologies and help small businesses participate in drug development, which is often dominated by large, established pharmaceutical companies.

SBIR/STTR has programs at 12 federal agencies that are coordinated through America's Seed Fund (SBA, 2025). For health-related programs, HHS has an SBIR/STTR program at both NIH and the Centers for Disease Control and Prevention (CDC), although the NIH program is much larger as CDC only offers SBIR. NIH awards around 1,300 SBIR/STTR awards per year, with a fiscal year (FY) 2023 budget of more than $1.4 billion (NIH SEED, n.d.; America's Seed Fund, n.d.), compared with around 20 SBIR awards (America's Seed Fund, n.d.) and a FY 2023 budget of $15 million at CDC (Sorkin, 2023).

There are several advantages to the unique funding mechanism. In addition to providing nondilutive funding, SBIR/STTR grants can attract additional interest and investment (Lee et al., 2021; NASEM, 2023a), as well as provide access to resources to guide commercialization. For example,

Connecting Awardees with Regulatory Experts (CARE) is an interagency collaboration that connects the National Cancer Institute's (NCI's) SBIR awardees with regulatory experts at FDA who provide feedback on regulatory questions early in the development process. In comparison with other NIH research project grants (e.g., R01, R21), SBIR/STTR programs support commercialization planning, market assessment, and organizational development in addition to scientific research.

NIH has several SBIR/STTR grant programs located in ICs across the agency, and 24 of the 27 ICs provide funding to small businesses (SEED, n.d.). These programs are correlated with positive economic outcomes. A 2018 economic impact analysis of NCI SBIR/STTR phase II grant awards from 1998 to 2010 found that funded programs had yielded $26.1 billion in economic output nationwide and added over 100,000 new jobs in the United States (HHS, 2018). In survey responses, 89 percent of respondents agreed with the statement "The NCI SBIR/STTR program provided funding at a pivotal or critical moment for the small business" (HHS, 2018). However, this analysis did not attempt to identify the causal effect of the SBIR/STTR awards, such as whether those projects would have found other sources of funding and resulted in similar economic success without the SBIR/STTR program.

More rigorous evaluation of these programs is important, though difficult to develop. For example, a National Academies consensus study report on the NIH's SBIR and STTR programs noted that the committee requested NIH research grant scoring data to conduct an analysis similar to one published in 2017 on the Department of Energy's SBIR program, which found that "an early-stage award approximately doubles the probability that a firm receives subsequent venture capital and has large, positive impacts on patenting and revenue," (Howell, 2017, p. 1,136), but NIH declined to provide the requested data (NASEM, 2022a). Using a coarser measure to identify investments, the National Academies committee found "no statistically significant difference in outcomes between those firms that received an SBIR/STTR award on their first application and those that applied to the programs but were rejected during that application cycle" when controlling for growth potential (NASEM, 2022a, p.162). The authors noted that this result is largely consistent with the program's high selectivity and that the finding suggests that other applicants similarly positioned were able to attract other sources of funding (NASEM, 2022a).

Of note, much of the evidence consists of interviews, surveys, and case studies, and while compelling, this qualitative evidence limits the ability to determine causal effects of the programs. In addition, reporting is often inconsistent. For example, available data underestimate patents generated by SBIR/STTR awardees who are less likely to report these results back to NIH (NASEM, 2022a). Despite some data limitations, the committee found:

Although it is difficult to prove that SBIR/STTR funding affected the ability of these firms to develop and produce these important drugs and devices, the awardee firms have had better commercialization outcomes relative to firms that did not receive this funding. (NASEM, 2022a, p. 145)

SBIR/STTR programs have many success stories, but there is room for improvement. Specifically, NIH's SBIR/STTR programs have been criticized for having evaluation criteria that are too similar to those of R01 research grants and prioritize scientific merit over commercialization potential (Dutta et al., 2023; NASEM, 2022a). The programs could be more effective by focusing on high-risk areas that are not covered by academic grants or private investment. In addition, multiple National Academies reports have emphasized that the programs could do more to provide training, resources, and outreach to potential applicants from underrepresented or underserved groups (NASEM, 2015, 2022a). Finally, improvements are needed in reporting and monitoring to enable more effective evaluation in future.

Finding 5-1: SBIR/STTR programs have shown promise in providing nondilutive funding to advance the commercialization of promising medical products and technologies, although more evaluation is needed. The programs could have more impact by focusing on high-risk areas that are not covered by academic grants or private investment.

Advanced Research Projects Agency for Health

One agency that is explicitly tasked with conducting high-risk, high-reward research is ARPA-H. Established within NIH, ARPA-H was created in 2022 with the mission of "supporting the development of high-impact solutions to society's most challenging health problems" (ARPA-H, 2024). ARPA-H's mission is to accelerate better outcomes through the support of effective solutions that address major challenges.

Modeled after other *ARPAs*, such as the Defense Advanced Research Projects Agency (DARPA) and the Advanced Research Projects Agency-Energy (ARPA-E), ARPA-H funds program managers in CEO-like roles for an initial 3-year term to design and launch research contracts devoted to addressing specific research challenges (Congressional Research Service, 2022). Program managers are given a high-degree of autonomy to innovate, rather than relying on the peer-review process, which as discussed earlier in this chapter, may hinder high-reward innovation.

ARPA-H currently supports several initiatives related to drug development in areas of unmet need. For example, ARPA-H has a program focused on low-cost cell therapies, called Engineering of Immune Cells Inside the Body (EMBODY). As discussed in Chapter 4, while the technology for cell and gene therapies has advanced, the cost of paying for these therapies remains a barrier to innovation and addressing unmet need. Programs like EMBODY, if successful, could help address some of these challenges.

Although ARPA-H is meant to address large health challenges, it currently does not have programs that focus specifically on areas where there is a mismatch in innovation and disease burden and unmet need. Expanding ARPA-H programs in some of these disease areas outlined in Chapter 3, such as cardiovascular disease and chronic obstructive pulmonary disease (COPD), would help advance innovation in these areas. Furthermore, continuing to expand ARPA-H's programs on diagnostics and biomarkers could also provide support in important areas.

TARGETED PROGRAMS TO ADDRESS UNMET MEDICAL NEEDS

Since 1938, drug sponsors have been required to demonstrate that their products are safe before marketing. However, it was not until 1962 that Congress added a requirement that drugs also be shown to be effective for their intended use. That year, in response to the thalidomide tragedy in Europe, Congress passed the Kefauver-Harris Drug Amendments to the Federal Food, Drug, and Cosmetic Act, which revolutionized drug regulatory standards in the United States (Greene and Podolsky, 2012; Meadows, 2006). Since adoption of these amendments, manufacturers have been required both to demonstrate that new drugs are safe for use and to provide "substantial evidence" of effectiveness through "adequate and well-controlled clinical investigations" before FDA may legally grant approval.[1] These preapproval safety and effectiveness requirements are critical to FDA's role in information production and innovation (Eisenberg, 2007; Kapczynski, 2018). By standing as a gatekeeper to the market—and to associated profits—FDA ensures that sponsors produce the essential information that patients and their clinicians need to guide decisions about treatment, including what drugs might be worth trying and which are not.

To develop drugs that are both safe and effective, it is essential to understand underlying disease mechanisms.[2] For many diseases, however, this fundamental information is lacking, contributing to unmet need. For example, despite billions of dollars spent by NIH to support research on Alzheimer's disease and related dementias (AD/ADRD), the underlying causes of AD/ADRD remain poorly understood (NASEM, 2024b). Until recently, pursuit of the amyloid hypothesis had limited success in drug

---

[1] New drugs, 21 U.S.C. 355 (2022).

[2] T. Zaks and M. Mackay. 2024. *Strategies to better align investments in innovations for therapeutic development with disease burden and unmet needs.* Presentation at committee meeting 2. June 18.

development, with ongoing debate about its scientific validity (Piller, 2022). FDA has granted accelerated approval to three monoclonal antibodies for AD since 2021 based on their effectiveness in reducing amyloid (an as yet unvalidated surrogate endpoint) and has granted regular approval to two of these drugs, lecanemab and donanemab.

In trials, both drugs resulted in a statistically significant slowing of cognitive decline, but at a rate below the minimal clinically important difference— the slowing may be too small to be noticed by patients, families, or clinicians. In addition, these drugs come with risks of serious side effects, raising questions about "their scope of application, long-term consequences, and the effect of their use in people living with mixed dementia" (NASEM, 2024b, p. 13).

Furthermore, many diseases lack adequate diagnostic tools. Most diseases have better outcomes if treatment can be started earlier in disease progression, but many diseases are associated with long diagnostic processes that delay early interventions. Accurate diagnostics can also improve clinical trial outcomes through the recruitment of appropriate patient populations including those most likely to benefit and excluding those unlikely to respond to the therapy. With such tools for clinical research and development, therapeutics with greater clinical benefit for patients may be more likely to appear on the market. Complicating the management of AD/ADRD patients, a diagnosis of Alzheimer's disease is predominantly based on cognitive, behavioral, or personality changes, which can be difficult to measure accurately, and the presentations of disease can often be atypical (NASEM, 2024b). Although there has been some development of better biomarkers for AD/ADRDS, more research is needed to more accurately and quickly diagnose AD/ADRDS, which could lead to better selection of appropriate patient candidates for current therapeutics and provide insights into new therapeutic targets and candidate therapeutics.

As discussed later in this chapter, FDA exercises a great deal of regulatory flexibility to approve promising drugs that address unmet needs. Furthermore, without a strong understanding of the pathophysiology of disease, it is difficult to know what mechanisms to target, so drug development lags or clinical trials fail. Therefore, for most diseases with unmet needs, the problem facing patients is not that FDA is standing in the way of approving promising drugs, but rather that there is difficulty in identifying strong drug candidates. Therefore, more basic and translational research is necessary to better support drug development. This research would improve the quality of products brought to FDA for approval and of the treatment options ultimately available to patients.

Finding 5-2: Many of the current drivers contributing to the misalignment of innovation and investment with disease burden and unmet need are not within FDA's immediate control.

Finding 5-3: Addressing unmet clinical need sometimes requires novel diagnostic tests to characterize diseases and disease states. For example, novel drugs often depend on accurate diagnostics to identify who should receive the treatment.

Conclusion 5-1: Diagnostics to characterize and detect disease states are critical for developing innovative therapies, targeting therapeutics to those who will benefit, and ensuring that patients have access to therapeutics early enough in their disease progression for therapeutics to be effective, and they are an important component of addressing unmet clinical need. Further incentives for development of innovative and accurate diagnostic tests that are necessary for drugs that address unmet medical needs could help resolve the mismatch among therapeutic investment, disease burden, and unmet need.

Although FDA approval is far downstream from scientific discovery, the agency has taken many steps to address unmet therapeutic needs. These approaches broadly fall into three categories (Figure 5-2): (1) programs that FDA administers to encourage investment to address unmet need; (2) efforts to mitigate broad scientific challenges inhibiting progress in drug development to address unmet need; and (3) programs to facilitate and expedite development and review of drugs to address unmet needs. Notably, some of these efforts have been devised and implemented by FDA, and some reflect authorities specifically granted to FDA from Congress. Each of these categories and their respective programs are outlined in detail in the section below.

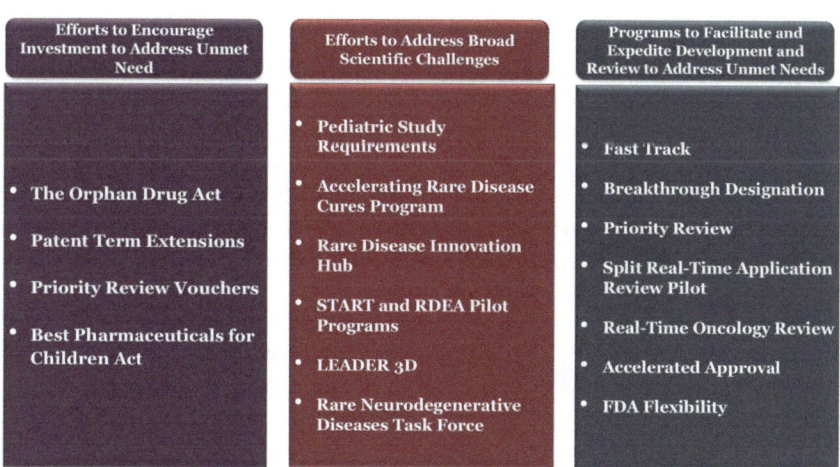

Efforts to Encourage Investment to Address Unmet Need	Efforts to Address Broad Scientific Challenges	Programs to Facilitate and Expedite Development and Review to Address Unmet Needs
• The Orphan Drug Act	• Pediatric Study Requirements	• Fast Track
• Patent Term Extensions	• Accelerating Rare Disease Cures Program	• Breakthrough Designation
• Priority Review Vouchers	• Rare Disease Innovation Hub	• Priority Review
• Best Pharmaceuticals for Children Act	• START and RDEA Pilot Programs	• Split Real-Time Application Review Pilot
	• LEADER 3D	• Real-Time Oncology Review
	• Rare Neurodegenerative Diseases Task Force	• Accelerated Approval
		• FDA Flexibility

FIGURE 5-2 FDA programs to address unmet needs.
NOTE: FDA = Food and Drug Administration.

Efforts to Encourage Investment to Address Unmet Need

In the past 3 decades, Congress has introduced programs intended to shape commercial drug development investments in accord with congressional and agency priorities. The following sections briefly summarize three existing incentives aimed at increasing drug development that exemplify programs intended to address the mismatch between investment and need.

As background to several of these incentives, it helps to first understand regulatory exclusivity, which is distinct from patent protection. To encourage innovation, FDA grants various exclusivities when approving new drug indications (FDA, n.d.). *Data exclusivity* prevents generic competition from relying on the original drug's clinical trial data in its own application for market approval. *Market exclusivity* completely blocks FDA approval of generic drugs even if the subsequent manufacturer conducts its own clinical trials. Owing to the cost of conducting clinical trials, in practice, data exclusivity has the same effect as market exclusivity in excluding most competitors (Congressional Research Service, 2017).

During the window of exclusivity, competitors are not able to bring generic drugs to market, allowing the brand-name drug an exclusive period in which to recoup its investment and secure profits, thereby encouraging investment in innovation. In most cases, for a new small-molecule drug with a new active moiety, companies are granted a new chemical entity (NCE) exclusivity of 5 years. Given the greater challenges of biologics development and manufacturing, new biologic medicines receive 12 years of exclusivity before biosimilar medicines may be marketed. In addition, there are distinct exclusivity periods specific to drugs to treat certain diseases or in certain populations. These exclusivity periods used for orphan drugs, antibiotic drugs, and pediatric populations have had varying success in promoting drug development in these areas.

Once exclusivity periods have expired (assuming patents have also expired), competitors are able to seek approval for generic or biosimilar versions of therapeutics, which generally reduce costs for patients. There are various incentives intended to promote generic and biosimilar competition (FDA, 2017). However, there are some therapeutics that never see lower costs for most patients, either because generics or biosimilars are never developed, or because lower-cost competitors fail to gain market share due to, for instance, efforts by brand-name manufacturers to maintain favorable formulary placement. Although outside of the scope of this committee, a recent Medicare Payment Advisory Commission report makes recommendations to ensure that once patents have expired, patients have access to cheaper therapeutics (MedPAC, 2023).

The Orphan Drug Act

The Orphan Drug Act (ODA) of 1983 was designed to address unmet medical needs by providing additional incentives for innovations for treating diseases with small markets. Under the original statute a rare disease was defined only as one designated by HHS as having "no reasonable expectation" that the development costs could be recovered from U.S. sales.[3] Because of administrative challenges obtaining this designation, the statute was amended in 1984 to provide the alternate definition of a disease that "affects less than 200,000 persons in the United States."[4] Drugs for diseases that meet either criteria are eligible for a tax credit for clinical trial expenses.[5] These tax credits were originally 50 percent but were reduced to 25 percent in 2017.[6] These drugs are also eligible for a 7-year period of FDA-administered market exclusivity (FDA, 2024c), which runs concurrently with new drug or biologic exclusivity, rather than being additive (Pharmaceutical Law Group, 2021). The ODA also provided HHS authority to make federal grants to cover certain costs of orphan drug development, including for clinical testing expenses incurred by private firms.[7] Generally, the market exclusivity is regarded as the most significant and important incentive offered in the ODA (IOM, 2010).

Consistent with other evidence that private firms respond to financial incentives, Yin (2008) estimates that this combination of incentives caused a 69 percent increase in the number of clinical trials for rare diseases. As he notes, however, some of these clinical trials for rare diseases may reflect rent-seeking, such as strategic relabeling of drug indications to fit rare disease categories. Yin's data also stop in 1994 and do not reflect more recent changes in orphan drug markets. Even without the ODA, orphan drugs have become attractive to develop because the path to regulatory approval for rare disease drugs has gotten shorter, cheaper, and generally more predictable than drugs for more common conditions. This is a result of the flexibility FDA shows to rare disease drugs both with regard to study design and approval standards and also regarding their eligibility for various expedited development pathways (discussed below).

There are also further reasons to believe that rare disease drug development would have improved even without the incentives offered in the ODA.

---

[3] Orphan Drug Act, 97-414. 97 (January 4, 1983).

[4] Designation of drugs for rare diseases or conditions, 21 U.S.C. 360bb (1985).

[5] Clinical testing expenses for certain drugs for rare diseases or conditions, 26 U.S.C. 45C (1983).

[6] An Act to Provide for Reconciliation Pursuant to Titles II and V of the Concurrent Resolution on the Budget for Fiscal Year 2018, Public Law 115-97, 115th Congress (December 22, 2017).

[7] Grants and contracts for development of drugs for rare diseases and conditions, 21 U.S.C. 360ee (1983).

Science—especially improvements in understanding human genetics—has enabled better understanding and development of treatment options for rare conditions. In addition, the prices of orphan designated drugs have soared, thereby increasing their profitability and making their return on investment strong despite small patient populations. Between 2008 and 2021, launch prices for orphan designated drugs were approximately seven times higher than for nonorphan drugs (Rome et al., 2022), and U.S. payers have typically been willing to cover effective therapies with higher prices for small patient populations (at least until the recent round of multimillion dollar therapies entering the market challenged even that model). Therefore, the two categories were both lucrative for manufacturers.

It is possible that orphan drugs have been, in some instances, as profitable for manufacturers as nonorphan drugs because of the incentives offered in the ODA. Furthermore, in some instances where the drug was not initially intended for orphan indications, ODA incentives can yield clinical trials resulting in labeling changes rather than providers prescribing these agents off-label. However, evidence shows that orphan exclusivity has had less of an effect over time. Between 1985 and 2014, orphan exclusivity rights outlasted the drug's last expiring patent in fewer and fewer cases: 50 percent for drugs approved in 1985–1994; 35 percent for drugs approved in 1995–2004; and 18 percent for drugs approved in 2005–2014 (Sarpatwari et al., 2018). Furthermore, the ODA has been subject to gaming in numerous ways. For example, in some cases, the ODA incentives have been applied to drugs beyond the goals of the legislation, including "for drugs that were not new, that were used broadly off-label beyond the FDA-approved rare disease indication, or that reached blockbuster sales despite the intent of the legislation to provide extra incentives for drugs for rare diseases that might not have been otherwise brought to market."[8]

Because the ODA's incentives have been so generous and may not currently be the driving force behind development of therapeutics in the rare disease space, and because they may be driving resources away from other important projects that are less financially attractive, there may be reason to narrow the ODA's incentives. For example, commentators have suggested that ODA incentives should be limited to areas in which there are no companies already in a disease space, rather than emphasizing a numeric patient threshold (Thomas and Caplan, 2019). Others have suggested terminating ODA incentives (or requiring clawback) when firms reach a revenue threshold (Bagley et al., 2019; Sinha et al., 2024), increasing regulatory scrutiny (Daniel et al., 2016), or allowing Medicare to negotiate prices for orphan drugs (Vogel et al., 2024a).

---

[8] Personal communication, A. S. Kesselheim, PORTAL (Program on Regulation, Therapeutics, and Law), January 3, 2025.

Finding 5-4: Whether or not the ODA is narrowed or otherwise adjusted, there is no convincing evidence to suggest that the recent growth in rare disease innovation is a result of ODA incentives.

Patent Term Extensions

Patent term extensions (PTEs) have been widely used since they were created by the Drug Price Competition and Patent Term Restoration Act of 1984 (also known as the Hatch-Waxman Act).[9] In general, a patent's term expires 20 years from when the patent application is filed (or 17 years from issuance for patents filed before June 8, 1995). Because pharmaceutical patents are typically filed early in the development process, before beginning clinical trials, many years of patent term often occur during the time spent completing clinical trials and obtaining FDA approval. Under the PTE statute, 35 U.S.C. § 156, drug developers may partially restore this lost term.[10] A developer may select one patent per approved drug to receive a PTE that restores term lost to FDA review and one-half of term lost to clinical testing. The statute also limits PTE to a maximum of 5 years of extension or 14 years total effective term after FDA approval. The developer applies for PTE with the U.S. Patent and Trademark Office, which then relies on FDA to determine the applicable extension period (Department of Commerce, 2021).

Lietzan and Lybecker (2020) examined PTE grants from 1984 through 2018 and found an average term restoration of about 3 years, resulting in an average effective patent exclusivity period of approximately 13 years (Lietzan and Lybecker, 2020). Because term restoration is only partial, they also found that effective patent life including PTE was still shorter for drugs with longer development times. The current PTE statute thus only partially addresses the problem of underinvestment in drugs that require long clinical trials, such as early-stage cancer treatments and preventatives (Budish ct al., 2015).

Some scholars have proposed more substantial adjustments to the patent term to address distortions in innovation incentives, including adjustments based on information about a drug's value that is obtained after the initial patent application (Buccafusco and Masur, 2021; Sukhatme and Bloche, 2019). While these policy proposals could in theory better align R&D investments with disease burden and unmet needs, the committee focused on other policy instruments for reforming the expected reward for bringing a new drug to market.

---

[9] The Hatch-Waxman Act: A Primer (2025), https://www.congress.gov/crs-product/R44643.

[10] The Hatch-Waxman Act. Extension of patent term. https://www.law.cornell.edu/uscode/text/35/156.

Priority Review Vouchers

The priority review voucher (PRV) program was originally created by Congress in 2007 to encourage the development of treatments for neglected tropical diseases and was replicated for rare pediatric diseases in 2012 (Ridley, 2017). To qualify for a PRV, which shortens the timeline for review of a qualifying marketing application from the usual 10 months to 6 months, a sponsor's application must be for a drug or biological product that addresses a neglected tropical disease or rare pediatric disease (Ridley and Régnier, 2016). In addition, FDA awards a voucher for priority review to the applicant company upon approval, which can then be used for another product that would otherwise not have qualified for priority review or, alternatively, sold to another company to use for one of their applications. The price for a PRV has hovered around $100 million to $150 million per voucher (Armstrong, 2025a). The idea is that the value of these vouchers will encourage investment in neglected tropical diseases and rare pediatric diseases, without any outlay of government funds, though as will be discussed in Chapter 6, decreasing the timeline to review an application will inevitably require additional resources and staffing to avoid delaying review times elsewhere in the agency.

In the pediatric rare disease PRV program, 36 drugs were issued a PRV upon approval between 2017 and 2023. The median annual price for drugs that were issued a voucher was $788,705, and they generated revenues similar to those of other brand drugs (Liu and Kesselheim, 2024). In a separate study comparing the development of adult rare disease drugs (for which no PRV program exists) to pediatric rare diseases, no difference was found in the period 2012–2018 in the rate at which drugs eligible for PRVs were introduced into clinical testing, although a greater number of PRV-qualified drugs reached phase II development (Hwang et al., 2019a). In the decade after the launch of the tropical disease PRV program in 2007, the number of drugs with neglected tropical disease indications entering phase I trials did not substantially change from the prior decade, before the PRV program's initiation (Jain et al., 2017).

Despite the lack of increases in therapeutics, it is likely that the value of the PRV helped companies raise capital to fund some therapeutic development, as most investors report taking PRVs into account in their net present value calculations. However, when PRVs expanded from neglected tropical diseases to pediatric rare diseases, it became clear that the value of the PRV is tied to the number of vouchers available in the market. While originally estimated to be valued at $325 million per drug, vouchers are now being sold for $100 million, on average (Barrie, 2024; Kesselheim, 2020).

This tension between empirical evidence and investor experience was also evident in a recent Government Accountability Office (GAO) report evaluating FDA's PRV programs, released in 2020 (GAO, 2020). GAO found limited studies evaluating PRV programs, but the available evidence indicated that "the programs had little or no effect on drug development" (GAO, 2020). Yet, when GAO spoke with seven drug sponsors for the report, all of them stated that "PRVs were a factor in drug development decisions." Another consideration is that in an earlier GAO report evaluating PRVs for pediatric rare diseases, FDA officials raised concerns about their ability to set public health priorities because the PRV program requires FDA officials to give priority reviews to new drug applications that would not otherwise qualify (Armstrong, 2025b). As of the writing of this report, the rare pediatric disease PRV program has not been renewed by Congress and began to sunset on December 20, 2024 (FDA, 2024i). The effect of not reauthorizing the rare pediatric PRV program will eliminate any new designations, and those companies with existing designations will only have until September 30, 2026, to gain marketing approval in order to earn the voucher.

> Finding 5-5: Without taking a position on whether priority review voucher programs should be renewed, the committee finds no convincing evidence to suggest that they should be expanded as a tool to better match investment and unmet need.

Best Pharmaceuticals for Children Act

As discussed in Chapter 4, diseases for pediatric populations and their remedies have long been understudied, leaving pediatricians to make decisions about drugs without the necessary information on proper dosage, efficacy, and safety. To incentivize research in pediatric populations, Congress passed the Best Pharmaceuticals for Children Act (BPCA) in 2002.[11] BPCA functions by providing an incentive for sponsors to conduct pediatric studies for products that have FDA approval but for which there are no data on the drug's use in children.

For drugs that are still on patent, sponsors get an additional 6 months of marketing exclusivity if they voluntarily conduct clinical studies in pediatric populations. Sponsors can either apply to the FDA for this extension, or FDA can make written requests to sponsors to complete the studies.

For drugs that are off patent, the responsible agency for implementing this program shifts from FDA to NIH. The Eunice Kennedy Shriver National Institute for Child Health and Human Development (NICHD) creates a list of priority medications to study in pediatric populations. NICHD then puts out a request for proposals for investigators to conduct

---

[11] *Best Pharmaceuticals for Children Act*, Public Law 107-109, 107th Congress (Jan. 4, 2000).

pediatric studies in the medications listed and provides funding for investigators to complete the studies.

BPCA (especially in coordination with the Pediatric Research Equity Act, discussed below) has been effective in getting studies to be conducted in pediatric populations, studies that resulted in over 60 labeling changes between 1998 and 2018 (Bourgeois and Kesselheim, 2019). The incentives offered through the BPCA have been particularly effective in getting research networks set up and getting clinical trials started in pediatric populations (NASEM, 2024a). However, there are some challenges to the BPCA. First, the studies are slow, taking on average 7 years from the time of FDA approval to complete studies in pediatrics (Carmack et al., 2020). This is partially because, as discussed in Chapter 4, pediatric trials can be expensive and difficult to recruit, especially once a product is on the market. Second, BPCA offers a blanket 6-month extension of exclusivity, which means that products that are popular in adult populations benefit from the incentive more than products that may benefit children more. And, third, research shows that sponsors tend to delay their request to FDA to conduct studies in pediatric populations until the end of their patent exclusivity, which delays the time it takes to complete the studies and have a labeling change (Olson and Yin, 2018).

Despite these challenges, BPCA works as a model for conducting research in populations that are understudied and for which there is little financial incentive to conduct research. A recent National Academies report called to expand the BPCA model (with some updates) to pregnant and lactating populations (NASEM, 2024a). However, BPCA works better as a model for incentivizing research with specific populations than incentivizing research on specific disease areas of high burden and large unmet need.

Conclusion 5-2: The committee did not find sufficient evidence to recommend expansion of priority review vouchers, orphan drug exclusivity, or patent term extensions in their current form to support drug development to better meet unmet needs.

Efforts to Address Broad Scientific Challenges

In addition to efforts to encourage investment, FDA has undertaken a variety of initiatives to mitigate scientific barriers to drug development in areas of unmet need—barriers ranging from insufficient incentives to pursue data in certain populations, to a lack of appropriate endpoints that could speed trials, to the need for close collaboration with regulators to ensure that scientific standards can be satisfied in challenging areas. Several of these initiatives, each of which demonstrates FDA's commitment to creatively addressing unmet need, are described below.

Pediatric Study Requirements

Following the passage of the BPCA in 2002, FDA issued an advance notice of proposed rulemaking to update the existing "pediatric rule" to require pediatric labeling changes for new drugs and devices.[12] However, a U.S. district court ruled several months later that the proposed rule exceeded FDA's statutory authority and enjoined FDA from enforcing the rule.[13] In response, Congress passed the Pediatric Research Equity Act (PREA) in 2003, which granted FDA the authority to require that sponsors conduct pediatric studies for new drugs and devices in pediatric populations before receiving FDA approval in the adult population.[14] Sponsors can request a waiver for conducting the required pediatric studies. If the product receives FDA approval before the waiver is denied, FDA requires that the studies be conducted as postmarketing studies (FDA, 2005).

PREA has been successful in getting dosage, safety, and efficacy data to be generated for pediatric populations. From the time it was enacted in 2003 until 2018, PREA resulted in 532 labeling changes, more than the BPCA (Bourgeois and Kesselheim, 2019). However, it does have some limitations. For one, PREA only requires that pediatric studies be conducted for the same indication under review for the adult population. Even if evidence indicates that a drug could be effective in treating a pediatric condition that differs from the adult indication, FDA does not have the authority to require that these studies be carried out (an exemption has been made for pediatric cancer treatment candidates) (Bourgeois and Kesselheim, 2019). Another limitation is that because pediatric studies take time to complete, FDA often grants sponsors deferrals to complete pediatric studies to expedite access for the adult population (Bourgeois and Hwang, 2017). This means that many new products are on the market for years (a median of 7 years) before pediatric labeling is updated (Hwang et al., 2019b).

Although PREA could be updated to address some of these limitations, it has been successful in generating pediatric labeling changes, especially when considered in combination with the BPCA.

Accelerating Rare Disease Cures Program (ARC)

In May 2022, FDA's Center for Drug Evaluation and Research (CDER) launched the Accelerating Rare disease Cures (ARC) program to

---

[12] Obtaining timely pediatric studies of and adequate pediatric labeling for human drugs and biologics, 67 FR 20070 (April 24, 2002).

[13] *Association of Amer. Phys. v. U.S. Food and Drug.* 226 F.Supp.2d 204. (U.S. District Court—District of Columbia, 2002).

[14] Pediatric Research Equity Act of 2003, S.650, 108th Congress (2003), https://www.congress.gov/bill/108th-congress/senate-bill/650.

advance research on drug development to address unmet needs of patients with rare diseases (FDA, 2024a). ARC is led by CDER's Office of New Drugs and is supported by CDER's dedicated rare diseases team. ARC brings together various FDA offices and programs, including the Center for Biologic Evaluation and Research (CBER), the Center for Devices and Radiological Health, the Oncology Center of Excellence, and the Office of the Commissioner.

ARC's scientific and regulatory initiatives focus on "strengthening platforms that facilitate natural history studies for rare diseases; developing, testing, and validating methodologies to construct novel endpoints; expanding the utilization of drug/disease modeling; establishing efficient approaches to dose selection for drugs for small population diseases; and expanding efforts in translational medicine approaches for individual rare disease programs" (FDA, 2024a, p. 10).

Rare Disease Innovation Hub

In 2024, FDA created the FDA Rare Disease Innovation Hub as a single point of contact, supporting intercenter collaboration, in an effort to "advance regulatory science with dedicated workstreams for consideration of novel endpoints, biomarker development and assays, innovative trial design, real-world evidence, and statistical methods" (FDA, 2024f; see also FDA, 2025c). To meet this goal, the hub plans to implement multipartner education and engagement opportunities that involve drug developers, FDA, patient organizations, other federal agencies (including NIH and ARPA-H), and researchers in support of education about novel approaches for the development of therapies for rare diseases (FDA, 2025e). There are up to three planned workshops in 2025, one of which is focused on designing clinical trials with a small and diminishing population of eligible trial participants. Furthermore, the hub seeks to encourage patient organizations and drug developers to engage in conversations throughout the drug development process. The hub is led by the directors of CDER and CBER and includes a steering committee of leadership from other centers and offices within FDA; its goal is to strengthen coordination and alignment among medical product centers through knowledge sharing. This is especially important given that one concern raised by rare disease drug developers has been a lack of consistency across agency centers and offices, with some exerting greater flexibility than others. Finally, the Rare Disease Innovation Hub is also intended to create a centralized point of contact for external partners.

START and RDEA Pilot Programs

In recent years, FDA has also created multiple pilot programs that seek to support the development of therapeutics to address unmet need for rare diseases.

One example is the pilot Support for clinical Trials Advancing Rare disease Therapeutics (START) initiative (FDA, 2024k). Launched in September 2023, START is a joint CDER and CBER effort open to sponsors of products that are in clinical trials under an active investigational new drug (IND) application. Eligible products for CDER are drugs intended to treat rare neurodegenerative conditions. Eligible products for CBER are gene or cell therapies intended to address an unmet medical need as a treatment for a serious rare disease or condition that is likely to lead to significant disability or death within the first decade of life (FDA, 2024k).

START has informally been described as "Operation Warp Speed" for rare diseases, in reference to the COVID era program that put industry and regulatory stakeholders in close collaboration to move drug development as quickly as possible by, in some instances, resolving barriers that limit efficiency and progress (Floersh, 2024). Sponsors selected to participate in START receive frequent advice and enhanced communication from FDA staff to address multiple potential drug development issues, including clinical study design, choice of control group and patient population, using nonclinical information, and product characterization (FDA, 2024k). Each of these issues can raise challenges for rare disease drug developers, especially given the small population sizes available for trial enrollment, associated statistical challenges, and open questions about the natural history of these diseases, which can make it difficult to select appropriate endpoints. Compounding these issues is that many rare disease drug developers are small companies without substantial prior experience or understanding of FDA requirements and expectations (Fernandez Lynch, 2023).

START's goal of active FDA engagement and timely responses is likely to help sponsors, particularly those who have less regulatory experience; speed drug development; and avoid issues that may later preclude regulatory approval. FDA already offers formal meetings to sponsors at several designated time points; however this process can take weeks or months, and decisions could be delayed or FDA-requested modifications could be difficult to accomplish within appropriate time frames. In contrast, through START's "more rapid, ad-hoc communications" with the agency (emails and videoconference responses), the program will provide a mechanism "to address development issues that would otherwise delay or prevent a promising novel drug from progressing" (Liang, 2024, p. 8) to the pivotal trial stage or to the stage at which sponsors meet with FDA immediately before submitting a marketing application (Eglovitch, 2024). While the START initiative will require substantial resources—and is currently limited to up to three participants for each center—it demonstrates FDA's goal of supporting the development of therapies for rare diseases that have unmet needs.

Similarly, the Rare Disease Endpoint Advancement (RDEA) pilot program, announced in October 2022, is designed to support novel efficacy endpoint development for drugs that treat rare diseases (FDA, 2022b). Also a joint CDER/CBER program, RDEA accepts sponsors with an active pre-IND or IND for a rare disease and sponsors without an active development program but planned natural history studies. The agency has also stated that it may consider accepting a proposal for a development program for a common disease that includes innovative or novel endpoint elements, including the specific endpoint or the methodology being developed, if there is sufficient justification that the proposal could be applicable to a rare disease. Furthermore, the proposed endpoint must be a novel efficacy endpoint intended to establish substantial evidence of effectiveness for a rare disease treatment. Given that RDEA is a pilot with limited resources, FDA states that one planned prioritization criterion is that the endpoint has potential to affect drug development more broadly, such as through a novel approach to develop an efficacy endpoint or an endpoint that could potentially be relevant to other diseases.

As both START and RDEA are pilot FDA programs, they will need additional resources to scale up and expand if they are to be successful.

LEADER 3D

The Learning and Education to Advance and Empower Rare Disease Drug Developers (LEADER 3D) initiative was also established to understand the challenges with bringing rare disease products to market (FDA, 2024g). LEADER 3D focuses on the development of educational content based on the needs of rare disease drug development stakeholders (FDA, 2025d). FDA's public report of an external stakeholder analysis as part of LEADER 3D includes multiple third-party recommendations to support rare disease drug development, including the following:

- address nonclinical challenges (e.g., resources about the use of nonanimal models),
- dose-finding (e.g., use of adaptive trial designs to determine dose selection),
- natural history studies and registries (e.g., development of educational materials highlighting when and how an external control group can be appropriately used in clinical trial design),

- novel endpoint and biomarker development (e.g., clarification about different types of endpoints and types of data expected to support regulatory approval),
- clinical trial design and analysis (e.g., materials to help sponsors identify when external data can replace or enhance control arms), and
- rare disease drug development regulatory considerations (providing more detailed information about using expedited programs for rare diseases) (FDA, 2024g).

Rare Neurodegenerative Diseases Task Force

The 2021 Accelerating Access to Critical Therapies for ALS Act was signed into law with the intention of advancing the understanding of neurodegenerative diseases and fostering development of treatments for amyotrophic lateral sclerosis (ALS) and other rare neurodegenerative diseases (FDA, 2021). This legislation provides (1) grants for research use of data from expanded access to ALS drugs, which have begun to be awarded; (2) a new public–private partnership to advance understanding of neurodegenerative diseases and foster development of treatments, which was announced in 2022 as the Critical Path for Rare Neurodegenerative Diseases; (3) a required 5-year FDA action plan to foster drug development and facilitate access to investigational drugs for ALS and other neurodegenerative diseases, which has already been published; (4) an FDA rare neurodegenerative disease grant program to be administered by the Office of Orphan Products Development focused on characterizing these diseases and their natural history, identifying molecular targets, and improving clinical development through use of innovative trial designs and trial networks; and (5) a GAO report to Congress analyzing both of the law's grant programs (FDA, 2022a; Fernandez Lynch, 2023).[15]

FDA's action plan for this legislation also includes an ALS science strategy to address challenges to ALS drug development, focused on improving characterization of ALS disease pathogenesis and natural history, facilitating access to investigational new drugs (such as through use of decentralized trial designs), enhancing clinical trial structure and agility, encouraging the incorporation of expanded access into clinical development programs, facilitating data sharing, and exploring innovative trial designs including novel statistical approaches for small populations (FDA, 2022a).

---

[15] Accelerating Access to Critical Therapies for ALS Act, HR 117-207, 117th Congress (2025). https://www.congress.gov/congressional-report/117th-congress/house-report/207/1.

Finding 5-6: Because FDA programs to address broad scientific challenges, with the exception of pediatric study requirements, have only been in place for a few years, it will be important to carefully evaluate their effect and resource burdens, both individually and collectively, and to devote additional resources to successful programs.

Programs to Facilitate and Expedite Development and Review to Address Unmet Needs

Expediting drug development and review may result in more drugs being brought to market more quickly. FDA has already established several expedited programs for drugs intended to address unmet need, which use a variety of tactics, including increased opportunities to meet with FDA throughout drug development, acceptance of alternative endpoints to speed clinical trials, and efforts to speed FDA's review of submitted applications (or portions thereof). Given the potential of these programs to signal a drug's promise, associated designations may encourage investment, particularly for precommercial companies (Hoffmann et al., 2019), in some ways acting also as an incentive.

Notably, FDA's expedited programs are being used with increasing frequency. For example, in 2024, 22 of CDER's 50 drug approvals (44 percent) used one or more of these expedited programs (FDA, 2025b).

Fast Track

FDA's fast track designation is available to drugs that are intended to treat a serious or life-threatening condition and that demonstrate the potential to address an unmet medical need (FDA, 2024d). The designation offers two important benefits. First, sponsors of fast track designated drugs are eligible for more frequent meetings, as well as written communication, with the FDA with the goal of discussing the drug's development plan to ensure that appropriate data are collected to support approval, as well as about the design of proposed clinical trials and the use of biomarkers (FDA, 2024d). Second, fast track designated drugs may receive rolling review, under which completed sections of a Biologic License Application (BLA) or New Drug Application (NDA) can be submitted for review as they become available, allowing concerns to be identified early and expediting the review process (FDA, 2024d).

Breakthrough Therapy Designation

The breakthrough therapy designation is available to drugs that are intended to treat a serious condition and for which preliminary clinical evidence indicates that the drug "may demonstrate substantial improvement over available therapy on a clinically significant endpoint(s)" (FDA, 2018a). Clinically significant endpoints are those that indicate an effect on irreversible morbidity or mortality or on symptoms that represent serious consequences of a given disease; these can include established surrogate endpoints, a surrogate or intermediate clinical endpoint considered reasonably likely to predict a clinical benefit; a pharmacodynamic biomarker that does not meet criteria as an acceptable surrogate but strongly suggests the potential for a clinically meaningful effect, and an improved safety profile compared to available therapy, with evidence of similar efficacy.

Receiving the breakthrough therapy designation means that the drug is eligible for all fast track designation features (i.e., more frequent interactions with FDA and rolling review), as well as intensive guidance on an efficient drug development program as early as phase I and organizational commitment involving senior FDA managers (FDA, 2024b). From 2013 to 2023, of 157 original indications approved by FDA with breakthrough therapy designation, 52 (33 percent) were granted accelerated approval and 105 (67 percent) traditional approval (Mooghali et al., 2024b). Among the traditional approvals, 61 (58 percent) were based on surrogate markers as primary endpoints.

One peer-reviewed study found that use of the breakthrough therapy designation reduced late-stage clinical development time by approximately 30 percent for new molecular entities (NMEs) (Miller et al., 2024). Of note, the effects on reducing clinical development time were stronger among privately held drug developers; the authors wrote that this highlighted the benefits of the breakthrough therapy designation on "smaller (or less resourced) drug developers on bringing these drugs to market" (Miller et al., 2024, p. 1,008). Furthermore, the authors estimated that the 30 percent reduction would lower the threshold needed for the NMEs to achieve profitability by 9–18 percent (Miller et al., 2024).

Important concerns regarding the breakthrough therapy designation have also been raised, however. As Darrow outlined in an initial evaluation of the program published in 2018, new drugs may be able to "meet technical requirements for the designation, and then be approved, despite having only modest efficacy" raising concerns that the designation may mislead patients who would reasonably expect breakthrough-designated drugs to be true clinical breakthroughs (Darrow et al., 2018).

Shortened Review Programs

Priority review Drugs may also receive a priority review designation from FDA if they are expected, if approved, to offer "significant improvements in the safety or effectiveness of the treatment, diagnosis, or prevention of serious conditions when compared to standard applications" (FDA, 2018b). Priority review designation means that FDA intends to take action on an application within 6 months, as compared to 10 months during a standard review (FDA, 2024e). Therefore, priority review can speed drugs to market by approximately 4 months, which is important for patient access and for sponsor profits. However, it should be noted that in practice, this did not lead to a significant difference in median clinical development time for fast track designation (6.6 years [4.2–9.3] years; $p = .10$) compared with clinical development for drugs that did not use an expedited program (7.2 [(5.3–9.5] years) (Wong et al., 2023).

Separately, as discussed above, some drug sponsors have been able to obtain priority review vouchers (after receiving approval for a drug for neglected tropical diseases and pediatric rare diseases), which can be sold to sponsors of drugs that would not otherwise be eligible for priority review, although with the lack of reauthorization by Congress at the end of 2024, its effect will be limited to those sponsors who have already secured a designation. Similarly, the PRV program for medical countermeasures has also sunset as of October 2023 and not been reauthorized by Congress (FDA, 2025f).

It is important that rushing to meet regulatory deadlines does not lead to patient harm, especially as Downing et al. (2017) found that postmarket safety events are more common for drugs that were approved near their regulatory deadline. Given the shorter window for priority review, this is something to be wary of.

Split Real-Time Application Review pilot Similar to the rolling review mentioned above in the context of fast track designation, the Split Real-Time Application Review (STAR) pilot program "aims to shorten the time from the date of complete submission to the action date, in order to allow earlier patient access to therapies that address an unmet medical need" (FDA, 2023). For efficacy supplements across all therapeutic areas and review disciplines that meet specific criteria, accepted STAR applications are submitted in "a 'split' fashion" (two parts with components submitted no longer than 3 months apart). The STAR pilot applies to supplemental drug and biologics applications proposing new uses of approved therapies to address unmet medical need when clinical evidence indicates the drug may demonstrate substantial improvement on a clinically relevant endpoint over available therapies. FDA will begin to review data once it receives a part 1 submission including, among other things, all components of the efficacy supplement except for final clinical study reports. The sponsor must then submit clinical study reports and integrated summaries of safety and effectiveness as a part 2 submission within 3 months. Because FDA will begin reviewing the data sooner, decisions will ideally move more quickly.

Real-Time Oncology Review   Launched in February 2018, the Real-Time Oncology Review (RTOR) does the following:

> aims to provide a more efficient review process to ensure that safe and effective treatments are available to patients as early as possible, while improving review quality and engaging in early iterative communication with the applicant. RTOR facilitates earlier submission of topline efficacy and safety results, prior to the submission of the complete application, to support an earlier start to the FDA's evaluation of the application (FDA, 2024j).

RTOR applies only to oncology drugs that are likely to demonstrate substantial improvements over available therapy or that meet criteria for expedited programs, that have straightforward study designs, and that have endpoints that can be easily interpreted (e.g., overall survival, response rates). RTOR does not affect the likelihood of approval, but FDA guidance states that "the intent of RTOR is to provide FDA reviewers earlier access to data, to identify data quality and potential review issues, and to potentially enable early feedback to the applicant, which can allow for a more streamlined and efficient review process" (HHS, 2023).

Research has found that one-fifth of new FDA oncology indication approvals from the 2018 inception of RTOR through December 31, 2023, came through RTOR (Mooghali et al., 2024a).

Regulatory flexibility

FDA has both formal and informal mechanisms for using regulatory flexibility to expand patient access to therapeutics, particularly for patients with unmet needs. This section reviews the formal process for flexibility, known as accelerated approval, as well as informal FDA flexibility that applies to both accelerated approval products and products receiving regular approval. The section ends with some of the challenges and limitations with these flexible approval standards.

Accelerated approval In response to the HIV/AIDs epidemic, FDA developed the accelerated approval program in 1992 to expedite approval for therapeutics that showed promise for treating serious conditions with unmet needs (Vereshchagina, 2022). In 2012, Congress codified this program into law in Section 901 of the Food and Drug Administration and Safety Innovation Act.[16] In contrast with FDA's other expedited programs,

---

[16] Food and Drug Administration Safety and Innovation Act, Public Law 112-144, 112th Congress (July 9, 2012).

accelerated approval is the only one that alters the type of evidence accepted for approval. Rather than clinical endpoints, which evaluate how patients feel, function, or survive, accelerated approval drugs meet the "substantial evidence" of effectiveness standard based on unvalidated surrogate endpoints or intermediate clinical endpoints other than irreversible morbidity or mortality that are deemed reasonably likely to predict clinical benefit. These surrogate endpoints, such as reduction in tumor size, often can be measured earlier than direct clinical benefits, such as survival. To confirm the predicted benefit, sponsors of accelerated approval drugs are required to complete postmarket trials on a mutually agreed upon timeline. If benefit is not confirmed, FDA may then use an expedited process to withdraw approval or change the label indication.

Use of the accelerated approval pathway is increasing, and between 1992 and 2021 there were 278 drugs granted accelerated approval (Beakes-Read et al., 2022). Most of these were for novel oncology drugs, but other nononcology drugs have also used this pathway (NASEM, 2023b). Furthermore, as noted in a recent National Academies report on rare diseases:

> Although the accelerated approval pathway is not used as frequently for nononcology rare diseases as it is for rare types of cancers, if applied appropriately, it can be a beneficial tool for bringing safe and effective drugs to patients who suffer from serious and life-threatening conditions and for whom there are no meaningful alternative treatment options. (NASEM, 2024c, p. 65)

Accelerated approval has recently been used for drugs to treat Alzheimer's disease, ALS, and Duchenne muscular dystrophy; FDA leadership has indicated that this pathway will become the norm for gene therapies (Brennan, 2024).

This increased use is because the accelerated approval pathway shortens clinical development times. Research examining 367 therapeutics approved by FDA between 2015 and 2022 found that clinical development times for drugs that used no expedited program were a median of 7.2 years (interquartile range 5.3–9.5) (Wong et al., 2023). However, approvals using accelerated approval had significantly shorter clinical development times: a median of 4.9 years, (4.0–7.4), with $p < .001$).

While accelerated approval has often been successful in getting innovative and effective drugs to patients more quickly than would otherwise have been possible, there are important concerns about the program. These have to do with the acceptance of controversial surrogate endpoints to support accelerated approval (Gyawali et al., 2019), using accelerated approval to "rescue" drugs that failed to meet clinical endpoints in pivotal trials (HHS, 2025), poor rigor and delay in confirmatory studies (HHS,

2025), challenges withdrawing drugs that fail to confirm benefit (Beakes-Read et al., 2022), conversion to regular approval despite not meeting endpoints in confirmatory studies (Joseph, 2024), and high prices (and coverage costs) without demonstrating benefit (Fashoyin-Aje et al., 2022; Liu et al., 2024). Because of these challenges, FDA and Congress have taken a number of steps toward addressing concerns about postmarket evidence generation and regulatory actions. In 2022, the Food and Drug Omnibus Reform Act was passed, which confirmed FDA's authority to require confirmatory studies to be underway prior to granting accelerated approval, required confirmatory study terms to be set by the date of accelerated approval, increased the frequency of progress reports on confirmatory studies, and adjusted the process for involuntary withdrawal.[17] For its part, FDA is increasingly requiring confirmatory studies to be underway before accelerated approval is granted (FDA, 2025a), which has been demonstrated to speed both conversion to regular approval and withdrawal depending on study outcome (Fashoyin-Aje et al., 2022). FDA has also taken more frequent action toward withdrawing approval following confirmatory studies that fail to demonstrate benefit. However, the balance between premarket and postmarket evidence generation remains challenging.

FDA flexibility Although not a formal expedited program, it is important to acknowledge that the FDA has increasingly employed substantial regulatory flexibility for most drug approvals, beyond the programs described above. For the purposes of this report, regulatory flexibility means the acceptance of weaker or less evidence in support of drug approval or less certainty about the effectiveness or clinical benefits of an approved drug indication. For example, a study of 273 new drugs and biologics approved by the agency for 339 indications over three periods (1995–1997, 2005–2007, 2015–2017) found that more recent approvals were based on fewer pivotal trials and that these trials were less rigorous (despite having longer durations) (Zhang et al., 2020). Another study found that 65 percent of drug approvals in 2022 were based on a single pivotal efficacy study (Kaplan et al., 2023). Johnston et al. (2023) also found that between 2018 and 2021, 10 percent of drugs approved by the FDA were based on pivotal studies with null findings for one or more primary efficacy endpoints. In practice, these statistics are exemplified by FDA's approval of Relyvrio, a drug for ALS that received FDA approval based on a single positive phase II trial (and was withdrawn when a phase III trial required by the European Medicines Agency failed to show benefit), and Elevidys, the first gene

---

[17] Food and Drug Amendments of 2022, H.R.7667, https://www.congress.gov/bill/117th-congress/house-bill/7667.

therapy for Duchenne muscular dystrophy, which received both accelerated and regular approval despite failure to meet primary endpoints (Feuerstein and Garde, 2024; Abrams et al., 2025).

Although regulatory flexibility can be appropriate, especially for rare diseases, it is important that the associated uncertainty be rapidly resolved. However, unlike the accelerated approval pathway, when FDA exercises regulatory flexibility outside that context, it does not require confirmatory studies, potentially leaving important gaps in understanding. It is imperative that this shortcoming in regulatory flexibility be resolved, although there has been neither regulatory nor congressional action to achieve this outcome (Fernandez Lynch et al., 2023).

> Finding 5-7: FDA currently exercises a great deal of regulatory flexibility both within and beyond existing programs and sometimes extends this flexibility too far by approving drugs that are unlikely to—or fail to—confirm benefit.

> Finding 5-8: Given the remaining unmet need, FDA is under pressure to increase regulatory flexibility beyond current approaches.

Challenges with flexible approval standards   One of the challenges with approaches that rely on postmarket evidence generation to confirm a drug's benefit after approval is that it can be difficult to encourage patients to enroll in rigorous studies once drugs become commercially available. Although adjusting payer coverage when drugs have not yet confirmed meaningful clinical benefit could help encourage participation, that approach has been politically unpopular to date (Fernandez Lynch and Bateman-House, 2020; Greenberg et al., 2025). As a result, confirmatory studies, when required, are often single-arm, conducted in patients outside the approved indication, or conducted outside the United States; they are also often delayed, as noted above (Dyachkova et al., 2024; Fernandez Lynch and Bateman-House, 2020; IQVIA, 2019). To the extent that FDA continues to rely on regulatory flexibility to approve drugs intended to meet unmet need, it is essential to explore additional steps to ensure that postmarket studies can be conducted quickly and well (Fernandez Lynch and Bateman-House, 2020).

Another challenge is that keeping pace with postmarketing requirements and enforcing these requirements requires the agency to have appropriate resources and staff. Beyond postmarketing requirements, to maintain and potentially expand the pathways and initiatives to address unmet needs outlined in this section requires resources and staff with the necessary expertise. Chapter 6 provides more details, but a well-resourced regulatory environment is needed for FDA to continue these programs.

Finding 5-9: Through a wide range of programs, FDA has demonstrated creativity and commitment to supporting the science necessary for successful drug development and to providing regulatory support for sponsors seeking to address unmet need, especially in the context of rare disease.

Finding 5-10: FDA has several programs designed to drive innovation in therapeutic areas of unmet need, including the breakthrough therapy and fast track designations, priority review, and accelerated approval, as well as less formal approaches to regulatory flexibility.

Conclusion 5-3: Additional resources are needed for FDA programs that successfully support endpoint development and validation, innovative trial design, and the resolution of other broad scientific challenges that impede drug development for unmet needs, as well as programs designed to support communication between sponsors and FDA to quickly resolve challenges arising in specific development programs.

Conclusion 5-4: Given important concerns about the accelerated approval pathway, recent adjustments need to be carefully monitored and further adjustments may be needed to promote rigor and confidence that accelerated approval drugs will, as quickly as is possible, confirm meaningful clinical benefit for patients or be withdrawn.

Conclusion 5-5: Current legislation and polices for FDA are sufficient to foster the approval of innovative drugs for unmet needs.

Conclusion 5-6: When traditional approval standards cannot be satisfied for scientific reasons, regulatory flexibility can be appropriate as long as the initial approval is based on a reasonable likelihood of clinical benefit and clinical benefit is rigorously and rapidly confirmed following approval.

Conclusion 5-7: Although patients facing serious unmet needs may reasonably be willing to accept greater uncertainty and risk, weak approval standards harm patients seeking clear information to guide treatment decisions, may impede the development of strong treatment options, and fail to incentivize investment in true innovation.

Conclusion 5-8: Support for innovation in the pre- and postmarket settings requires a well-resourced regulatory environment, including attracting and retaining FDA staff with the necessary experience and expertise.

PUBLIC–PRIVATE PARTNERSHIPS

Public–private partnerships (PPPs) could provide a mechanism for aligning public- and private-sector financial investments. PPPs have become instrumental in advancing drug development by combining the strengths of governmental bodies, academic institutions, and private industry. These collaborations are designed to accelerate the translation of scientific research into effective medical treatments, addressing complex health challenges more efficiently than traditional models.

PPPs can take both simple and complex formats. In their simplest form, partnerships between the public and private sectors can be bilateral agreements between two organizations. In the case of the federal government and the private sector, these take many forms depending on the type of partnership sought. Two examples of these bilateral agreements are targeted drug development grant programs, such as the Network for Excellence in Neuroscience Clinical Trials (NeuroNEXT) and the National Cancer Institute's (NCI) Experimental Therapeutics (NExT) programs, and cooperative research and development agreements (CRADAs). PPPs can also be complex, multistakeholder agreements that involve projects between government, industry, academia, and nonprofit organizations, such as the Accelerating Medicines Partnerships (AMP) and Operation Warp Speed (OWS).

Bilateral Agreements

Targeted Drug Development Grant Programs

Federal agencies often sponsor targeted drug development programs to provide directed resources to aid organizations in areas of the drug development process where smaller companies or nonprofits generally find it challenging to secure funding (HHS, 2018; SEED, n.d.). For example, NeuroNEXT is an initiative funded by the National Institute of Neurological Disorders and Stroke to facilitate phase II clinical trials for neurological diseases (NeuroNEXT, n.d.; NINDS, 2025). NeuroNEXT fosters collaborations among academia, private foundations, and industry partners, providing a centralized institutional review board (IRB) and standardized agreements to facilitate efficient trial initiation and management. An independent evaluation of NeuroNEXT in 2020 found that the program "successfully enrolled participants at or ahead of schedule, collected high-quality data, published primary results in high-impact journals, and provided mentorship, expert statistical and trial management support to several new investigators" (Cudkowicz et al., 2020, p. 3).

Another example is the NExT program, funded by NCI to advance the discovery and development of novel cancer therapies, particularly those not typically pursued by private industry. NExT accepts applications from various entities, including academic institutions, private companies, and government organizations. Proposals are evaluated based on scientific merit, feasibility, alignment with NCI's mission, novelty, and clinical need. Instead of providing direct funding, NExT offers access to NCI's extensive contract-based resources to support the development of accepted projects, depending on where the project is in development (NCI, n.d.-b). For example, a project in the early discovery phase can receive resources from the Frederick National Labs for Cancer Research or the Chemical Biology Consortium, which can assist with *in vitro* and *in vivo* target validation, high-throughput screening, biophysical characterization, and more (NCI, n.d.-a). Although the committee is unaware of any independent evaluations of the program, a 2021 presentation from the Deputy Director for Clinical and Translational Research at NCI shared that the program had led to over 50 publications, over 10 patents filed, and 10 U.S. and international patents awarded. Furthermore, at the time of the presentation (June 2021), five therapeutic agents had begun to be investigated in clinic trials and two therapeutics anticipated filing INDs that year.[18]

The Bridging Interventional Development Gaps (BrIDGs) program, run through NCATS, functions similarly to the NExT program (NCATS, 2024). The BrIDGs program provides contracting services to generate preclinical and clinical-grade material to use in IND applications to the FDA. Unlike NExT, which focuses on cancer projects, BrIDGs is not disease specific and can be used to advance high-risk therapies for both common and rare diseases.

Cooperative Research and Development Agreements

Established under the Federal Technology Transfer Act of 1986, CRADAs have become a vital mechanism for fostering public–private partnerships, driving innovation, and ensuring that federally developed technologies benefit society (NIH Office of Technology Transfer, n.d.). CRADAs are one of the most common bilateral agreements used by the United States federal government. A CRADA is a formal arrangement between a federal laboratory or research entity and a nonfederal entity, such as a private company, university, or nonprofit organization, to collaboratively conduct R&D in areas aligning with the federal agency's mission (Naval Postgraduate School, 2022). Some

---

[18] As of May 2025, it appears that one of the therapeutic agents anticipating an IND filing has moved into phase I and II trials; see https://clinicaltrials.gov/study/NCT04629443 (accessed May 23, 2025). A number of the agents already in clinical trials as of 2021 are still undergoing testing; see https://clinicaltrials.gov/study/NCT01273168 and https://clinicaltrials.gov/study/NCT04512235 (accessed May 23, 2025).

of the key features of partnerships under CRADAs include resource sharing, prenegotiated intellectual property (IP) rights, mutual confidentiality terms, and the ability for accelerated technology transfer and commercialization (Homeland Security Science and Technology, 2020; Naval Postgraduate School, 2022). For resource sharing, both parties can contribute in-kind resources; however, while the private-sector partner can provide the federal partner funding, the federal partner cannot provide the private-sector partner funding under the agreement (Naval Postgraduate School, 2022).

For IP rights, while every federal CRADA does have variations on the time point at which IP can be claimed, the nonfederal partner typically retains rights to inventions it develops under the CRADA and may be granted an option to negotiate exclusive or nonexclusive licenses for inventions developed jointly or by the federal laboratory, subject to government-use rights (EPA, 2024). These IP terms often also allow for disclosure of public release of information about the data and inventions generated (STIP, n.d.). While there any many examples of drug approvals that have resulted from CRADAs, there are some real successes for HER2+ breast cancer treatment developed using CRADAs between industry and NCI: Herceptin (trastuzumab) for adjuvant HER2+ early breast cancer and Perjeta (petuzumab) for neoadjuvant HER2+ early breast cancer (Romond et al., 2005).

Multistakeholder PPPs

While these two-party PPPs help to facilitate many aspects of drug development, especially for smaller organizations, tackling the challenges involved in creating therapeutics for areas of mismatch between unmet need/disease burden and innovation investment will often require larger, more complex PPPs. To create these partnerships, federal scientific agencies often call upon their congressionally mandated, affiliated nonprofit organization. Several U.S. government scientific agencies are supported by congressionally established nonprofit foundations, each created to advance its particular missions through PPPs. Box 5-2 provides an overview of some of these foundations, including the legislation that established them and their core missions.

More complex PPP formats facilitated by the organizations described above often involve multiple stakeholders across both the public and private sectors, including representatives from government, industry, academia, nonprofits, and organizations representing persons with lived experience, which requires more complex structures for funding and contracting. A few notable examples are the Foundation for the National Institutes of Health (FNIH) Biomarkers Consortium and the AMP, which are overseen by Operation Warp Speed (Box 5-3). The Biomarkers Consortium unites

BOX 5-2
Congressionally Mandated Nonprofit Foundations

Congress has established a number of agency-affiliated nonprofit research foundations to advance the research and development (R&D) goals of the U.S. government. The goals of these nonprofits are: "(1) providing a flexible and efficient mechanism for establishing public–private R&D partnerships; (2) enabling the solicitation, acceptance, and use of private donations to supplement the work performed with federal R&D funds; (3) increasing technology transfer and the commercialization of federally funded R&D; (4) improving the ability of federal agencies to attract and retain scientific talent; and (5) enhancing public education and awareness regarding the role and value of federal R&D" (Gallo and Hogue., 2022, p. i) These nonprofit organizations exist for federal agencies focused on health, agriculture, energy, and veterans. The text below describes several of the foundations focused on health.

Foundation for the National Institutes of Health (FNIH)
- Establishment: The FNIH was established by Congress in 1990 under Section 499 of the Public Health Service Act (42 U.S.C. 290b).[a]
- Mission: The foundation is intended to support NIH in its mission by facilitating public–private partnerships that advance biomedical research and the application of breakthrough discoveries to improve health (FNIH, 2025b).

Reagan-Udall Foundation for the Food and Drug Administration (FDA)
- Establishment: Created by Congress in 2007 through the Food and Drug Administration Amendments Act, the Reagan-Udall Foundation operates as an independent 501(c)(3) organization.
- Mission: The foundation's purpose is to advance the mission of the FDA by modernizing product development, accelerating innovation, and enhancing product safety.[b]

CDC Foundation
- Establishment: The CDC Foundation was established by Congress in 1992 as an independent, nonprofit organization to support the Centers for Disease Control and Prevention (CDC).
- Mission: The foundation helps CDC do more, faster, by forging partnerships between CDC and others to fight threats to health and safety (CDC Foundation, 2025).

continued

BOX 5-2 Continued

Henry M. Jackson Foundation for the Advancement of Military Medicine

- Establishment: The Henry M. Jackson Foundation for the Advancement of Military Medicine was established by Congress in 1983 (Jackson Foundation, 2025).
- Mission: The Henry M. Jackson Foundation partners to advance military medicine for the benefit of the nation's warfighters. In the original legislation, one of the foundation's core functions was to serve as a link between military researchers and the private medical sector (Jackson Foundation, 2025).

---

[a] Establishment and duties of Foundation, 42 U.S.C. 290b (1990). https://www.law.cornell.edu/uscode/text/42/290b.

[b] Food and Drug Administration Amendments Act. Public Law 110-85, 110th Congress (September 27, 2007).

BOX 5-3
Lessons Learned from the COVID-19 Pandemic

In response to the COVID-19 pandemic, the U.S. government created the public–private partnership Operation Warp Speed (OWS) (later renamed the Countermeasures Acceleration Group) to accelerate the development of vaccines, therapeutics, and diagnostics (D'Souza et al., 2024). The central premise of OWS was to advance purchase orders of vaccines to guarantee demand, while also providing financial support up front to aid in development costs. OWS pursued multiple candidates with varying technologies to expand the likelihood of success. Two of the vaccine candidates sponsored by OWS completed clinical trials in just 10 months, four of the candidates received Food and Drug Administration (FDA) emergency use authorization, and two of this later received full FDA approval (D'Souza et al., 2024).

The success of OWS in spurring development of these vaccines provides several lessons that are relevant to aligning innovation with unmet needs and disease burden (and also lessons on public health emergencies, which are beyond the committee's charge and not covered here). First, OWS invested in a high-risk technology—mRNA vaccines—that ultimately became the leading technology for COVID-19 vaccines

BOX 5-3 Continued

(D'Souza et al., 2024). As discussed earlier in this chapter, the National Institutes of Health (NIH) has been criticized for funding "safe" research projects that are not innovative enough to meet the unmet needs of the United States. However, the investments made by OWS, which were considered very high risk at the time, show that public investment in high-risk, high-reward technology can pay off. In fact, some of the speed and derisking of mRNA vaccines can likely be attributed to years of prepandemic public investment in developing the technology through the Biomedical Advanced Research and Development Authority and the Department of Defense (Lalani et al., 2023).

Second, OWS shows that public–private partnerships (PPPs) among government agencies, academia, and industry can be a successful way to pool resources and share expertise in therapeutic development (Correa-De Araujo et al., 2023; Reagan-Udall Foundation for the FDA, 2022). During the pandemic, FNIH set up a PPP called ACTIV (Accelerating COVID-19 Therapeutic Interventions and Vaccines), to better coordinate and accelerate research on COVID-19 therapeutics and vaccines. ACTIV was successful in setting a research agenda for COVID-19 counter-measures, which allowed for better resourced trials for necessary treatments. Furthermore, ACTIV was helpful in identifying specific disease endpoints and working with the various stakeholders to develop regula-tory guidance and ultimately accelerate product development (Keshtkar-Jahromi et al., 2024). Although it would not be feasible to develop a PPP with the priority that OWS had for every disease, the coordination that ACTIV provided could be replicated for other high-priority disease states.

Finally, many of the clinical trial networks that were set up in response to the COVID-19 pandemic built on existing public clinical trial infrastruc-ture set up by the National Institute of Allergy and Infectious Diseases (NIH, 2020; Reagan-Udall Foundation for the FDA, 2022). To expedite clinical trials for disease areas of high unmet need, or to prepare for another public health emergency, a clinical trial infrastructure that can be built and maintained would allow for more rapid engagement and for better efficiency instead of running smaller—and therefore likely less informative—trials. Considerations for sustainable clinical trial infrastruc-ture have been discussed in previous National Academies activities (IOM, 2012).

diverse stakeholders from all organization types noted above, including over 70 industry and nonprofit members, plus numerous academics for each project to identify and validate biomarkers and drug development tools for enhancing therapeutic development and regulatory decision making. Since it was formed in 2006, the consortium has made significant achievements in developing, validating, and qualifying biomarkers, including for metabolic disorders, cancer, and more. Such a model has evolved and can continue to evolve strategically to meet emerging scientific needs, especially in the areas of unmet need (Menetski et al., 2019).

The AMP programs are mostly PPPs created to develop large data-sets of multiparametric data for drug target identification and validation, engaging government, industry, academics, nonprofits, and persons with lived experience. Across the 10 AMP partnerships, there are 34 industry partners, 16 NIH institutes and centers, and 37 nonprofit organizations. Although there are not yet any drug candidates that originate from the AMP programs, they have potential benefits for drug development that are true of other PPPs, including:

1. Resource sharing: pooling of financial resources, expertise, and infrastructure from both public and private sectors, facilitating large-scale projects that might be unmanageable for individual entities;
2. Accelerated research: expediting the drug discovery process by combining scientific research capabilities with practical develop-ment and distribution expertise;
3. Risk mitigation: sharing the risks associated with drug develop-ment encourages investment in innovative research areas that may be too risky for individual private companies to undertake alone;
4. Standardization and data sharing: promoting the development of standardized protocols and open data sharing, enhancing reproduc-ibility and validation across the scientific community; and
5. Finally, critical for drug development, enhanced target valida-tion: validating biological targets for therapy jointly across a field increases the likelihood of successful drug development and reduces late-stage failures (Dolgin, 2019).

Given the goals of AMP, it is important to recognize that not all success-ful PPPs aim to advance a therapeutic to market. Some, such as AMP, aim to facilitate better selection of targets for treatment, which, as noted, can reduce late-stage failures and advance drug development in ways that are more dif-ficult to evaluate than just drug approvals. For example, the Type 2 Diabetes Knowledge Portal, supported by AMP, enables investigators to prioritize 18 targets, and importantly, deprioritize a further 30 (FNIH, 2024).

While most of AMP's work as described above is valuable for drug development, one of the AMP programs is also worth highlighting for how it is working in a different way to promote therapies in the area of unmet need of rare diseases. The AMP Bespoke Gene Therapy Consortium (BGTC), which launched on October 27, 2021, instead of seeking to identify and validate targets, is focused on accelerating the development of gene therapies for rare genetic diseases that typically lack commercial interest (NCATS, 2021). The consortium aims to create a comprehensive "playbook" for developing gene therapies, encompassing streamlined templates, master regulatory files, and uniform manufacturing processes. This playbook will be validated through up to eight clinical trial test cases, providing insights that can be used to streamline the regulatory process for future gene therapy development. By focusing on a single gene therapy platform—the adeno-associated virus vectors, known for their safety in gene delivery—BGTC seeks to make this technology more accessible for treating a broader range of diseases (FNIH, 2025a). Critical to this PPP is that not only researchers but regulators helped design the program and will also be part of its execution and management. In fact, work from this program helped to shape FDA's draft guidance on platform therapies (FDA, 2024h). This program demonstrates that PPPs can also assist with the shaping of regulatory policies for drug development, and not just discovery and clinical research.

Large complex PPPs have been used to improve the drug development pipeline in countries other than the United States. In Europe, the Innovative Health Initiative (IHI), formerly the Innovative Medicines Initiative, is a large-scale PPP designed to foster drug discovery and development. By pooling resources and expertise from public and private sectors, IHI addresses bottlenecks in pharmaceutical innovation, particularly in such areas as translational immunology and neuropsychiatric disorders. The initiative has made substantial progress, exemplified by several translational datacentric projects targeting Alzheimer's disease and other conditions (Goldman, 2012; Goldman et al., 2013).

PPPs are also playing a promising role in tackling global health issues, such as neglected diseases prevalent in low-income regions. Collaborations between public entities and private companies have revitalized research and development efforts in areas that were previously underfunded, leading to new treatments and improved health outcomes. The Global Health Innovative Technology (GHIT) Fund, established in Japan, is an international public–private partnership dedicated to advancing global health R&D. Its primary mission is to mobilize Japanese industry, academia, and research institutions to collaborate with global partners in creating new drugs, vaccines, and diagnostics targeting malaria, tuberculosis, and neglected tropical diseases. By investing in the development of health technologies, the GHIT Fund aims to deliver innovative solutions for diseases that disproportionately affect underserved populations. As one of the world's first public–private partnership fund for global health R&D, the GHIT Fund exemplifies a pioneering approach to funding and facilitating the development of essential health technologies (GHIT Fund, 2025).

> Finding 5-11: PPPs can effectively enable the private sector to share both costs and risks.

> Finding 5-12: Every scientific health research agency has a congressionally mandated nonprofit organization that could be useful in building PPPs.

Challenges with PPPs

Despite the successes of PPPs and the potential to expand them to enhance innovation in needed therapeutic areas, several barriers exist within the U.S. context to developing more PPPs. First, PPPs often spring from federal agencies wanting to expand therapeutic development in a specific area and approaching industry about entering a PPP to contribute financial support or in-kind resources and assets. In areas of high unmet need with low economic incentives for the private sector, these are often shelved assets or research concepts that companies have developed but chosen not to pursue. However, the federal agencies do not always have insight into what shelved assets or research exists and therefore are unable to approach companies about developing these assets. This limits the usefulness of PPPs, particularly for addressing topics of high unmet need.

Some companies exist with the sole purpose of seeking out abandoned assets from other companies and developing them. However, even for these companies, it is a time- and labor-intensive process to seek out these abandoned assets that show promise. While these companies fill a need in the market and have been successful developing drugs for pediatric oncology, autoimmune diseases, pulmonary diseases, and more, there are still gaps in the market for therapeutics that are either too high risk to be able to raise capital or that market dynamics still do not favor. For these drugs that remain shelved, despite therapeutic promise, PPPs could be useful in advancing these to market. FNIH is working with NCI and FDA Oncology Center of Excellence to create such a PPP that would create a resource network and process to develop drugs for ultrarare cancers with well-defined biological targets, but for which there is no economic incentive for industry, even small start-ups, to create therapies to treat. The partnership aims to either take shelved assets from companies that address known biological targets within these ultrarare cancers or develop novel agents directed at these well-defined biological targets. This PPP is just beginning its design phase and engaging all the necessary partners to create such a network, but it intends to launch pilot projects in 2026 (FNIH, 2025c).

Another potential barrier to advancing PPPs is the lack of an existing clinical trial infrastructure that is "warm" and ready to use at any time. As described in Box 5-3, this was one of the lessons of the COVID-19 pandemic, and having a network that is ready to use for the next public health emergency is critical for quickly developing innovative therapeutics. With the exception of the National Cancer Institute, many institutes within NIH will create infrastructure for a single clinical trial, run the clinical trial, and then, without sustainable funding to keep the networks active, will have to disband the work (Eisenberg et al., 2012). This process is both inefficient and expensive, and improving the process could benefit both the public and the private sectors. On the public side, having stable clinical trial networks to run trials as needed would save time and resources. On the private side, industry could use public networks to efficiently set up trials where there currently is not a strong market incentive to do so. For example, a network for rare disease trials could help incentivize industry to conduct trials in these populations. The need for better clinical trial infrastructure was a consistent theme in the National Academies' workshop on Envisioning a Transformed Clinical Trials Enterprise for 2030 (NASEM, 2022b). Advancing these networks are critical for advancing clinical trials in the current landscape.

Regardless of the type of PPP or the designated coordinating entity, it is critical to remember that the success of PPPs depends on clear governance structures, equitable sharing of risks and rewards, the expertise of staff to navigate the drug development ecosystem, and alignment of objectives among partners. Effective partnerships require transparent communication, mutual trust, and a shared commitment to public health goals. When managed well, PPPs can significantly enhance the efficiency and effectiveness of drug development pipelines, ultimately bringing innovative therapies to patients more rapidly. To manage these partnerships well takes resources, which can be a barrier for some smaller organizations to participate and enter into these PPPs. Some larger PPPs have managed this by offering a sliding scale of participation, tiered by the size of the organization and R&D budget. However, some organizations may find it difficult to contribute the required amount to benefit and share with others engaged in PPPs.

One thing that both the biomarkers consortium and the AMP PPPs demonstrate is that these more complex partnerships function best in the precompetitive space where no IP is claimed or else if all IP is jointly owned by the partnership. Large PPPs have a more challenging time operating if a single or even just a few partners are seeking to claim the work of the partnership and exclusively develop it for their own monetary gain. Because of this, it can be challenging to evaluate the success of PPPs, particularly when the goal of the PPP is in the precompetitive space. Often, some of the earlier work is conducted using the PPPs, with companies doing some of the later-stage trials, so it is difficult to track what has come to market solely because of PPPs. Further, some PPPS, like AMP, aim to advance more precise therapeutic targets by ruling out some potential targets to prevent investments in therapeutics that will ultimately fail in later stage trials.

> *Conclusion 5-9: Strengthening and expanding public–private partnerships, such as the Network for Excellence in Neuroscience Clinical Trials, the National Cancer Institute Experimental Therapeutics program, and Bridging Interventional Development Gaps, could help address innovation challenges for therapeutic areas with unmet needs.*

PRICING AND ACCESS

As reviewed in Chapter 4, financial considerations are critical to the discussion of R&D development in the pharmaceutical industry, including estimation of financial returns, which are related to expected market size and price per user (Lakdawalla and Sood, 2012). For example, evidence from Blume-Kohout and Sood (2013) and Dranove et al. (2020) highlight increased R&D activity for drug products with a high share of Medicare-eligible population following the enactment of Medicare's outpatient prescription drug benefit (Part D). Notably, Dranove et al. also found that the strongest and most immediate R&D response to Part D's passage was for clinical trials that represented less scientific novelty, with a more modest and delayed response for potential scientific breakthroughs.

Other empirical work on pharmaceutical markets similarly shows that firms respond to financial incentives by increasing R&D on products that are expected to receive larger returns (Vernon, 2005). For example, studies have demonstrated that increases in expected market size based on changing disease burden result in increased number of drugs targeting that disease (Acemoglu and Linn, 2004; Dubois et al., 2015), that increases in drug prices are associated with increased R&D intensity (Giaccotto et al., 2005), and that changes in policies of certain vaccines caused increases in the profitability of those vaccines (Finkelstein, 2004). Together, these results suggest that increasing the expected financial returns on certain products, through application of value-based prices and reimbursement policy that explicitly addresses unmet need, is likely to increase the R&D effort directed toward those products (Grabowski and Vernon, 2000). The following sections review different payers in the U.S. health care system, describe how pricing is currently determined in the United States, and review ways this could be adjusted to better incentivize innovation in areas of unmet need.

Finding 5-13: An expectation of increased financial return for a certain class of pharmaceutical product has been shown to increase R&D effort on those products.

Primary U.S. Payers

According to a 2023 survey, about 92 percent of people in the United States had health insurance for either some or all of the year (Keisler-Starkey and Bunch, 2024). About 65.4 percent of people with health insurance were covered by private health insurance, and 36.3 percent were covered by public coverage, mostly by either Medicaid or Medicare (Keisler-Starkey and Bunch, 2024).[19] Spending on medications varies across payers based on the demographic makeup of the populations they cover and the prevalence of conditions that the medications are used to treat. In addition, medication spending can ranges from outpatient pharmacy (retail sales) to clinician-administered drugs. There are limited comprehensive reports of the combined drug spending by payer, thus the focus here is on retail drug spending.

Medicare provides coverage to individuals 65 years of age or older, younger populations who qualify through Social Security disability insurance as meeting criteria for long-term disability, and those with either end-stage renal disease or amyotrophic lateral sclerosis. Medicare is the primary payer for drugs in the United States, accounting for a third of retail drug spending. Medicare is administered by the Centers for Medicare & Medicaid Services (CMS), which is therefore a critical body in the reimbursement of drug products in the United States (Cubanski et al., 2019).

Medicaid provides insurance coverage to low-income individuals, children, and pregnant/postpartum populations, and is jointly administered by the states and CMS. While outpatient prescription drug coverage is not one of the benefits required by the federal government for Medicaid, all states currently provide prescription drug benefits. Medicaid represents around 10 percent of U.S. drug spending.

Finally, private insurers represent around 40 percent of U.S. retail drug spending, though the private insurance market is segmented into individual market plans (sold directly to individual consumers), self-funded employer-sponsored plans, and fully insured employer-sponsored plans.

---

[19] These types of coverage are not mutually exclusive because people can be covered by multiple types of insurance over the course of a year; thus, the sum of private and public coverage can exceed 100 percent (Keisler-Starkey and Bunch, 2024).

U.S. Coverage and Reimbursement of Drug Products

In the United States there is no formal regulation of drug list prices, which are set freely by drug manufacturers. Though not the only factor, this results in prices that are higher than those in other similarly resourced countries with price regulation mechanisms, even after accounting for manufacturer discounts (Wouters et al., 2025). For every dollar that consumers in other countries pay for brand name drugs, the U.S. consumer pays $2.78 (Mulcahy et al., 2024). High prices and market size cement the United States as the largest contributor to the pharmaceutical market, accounting for about 50 percent of global sale revenues, but only 13 percent of volume (Parasrampuria and Murphy, 2024). The U.S. share of the market has only grown over time, with the total share of U.S. sales for prescription drugs increasing 23 percent from 2017 to 2022 (Parasrampuria and Murphy, 2024). One of the reasons the United States pays so much more for prescription drugs than other countries is likely its fragmented health insurance system, where coverage and reimbursement of drug products are variable across payers. This means that negotiations for drug prices are split across many different entities, which reduces the power of any one unit to negotiate drug prices. Moreover, because Medicaid and Medicare Part D tie reimbursements to private-sector prices, they create incentives for firms to raise prices for privately insured patients (Duggan and Scott Morton, 2006). Furthermore, prior to the Inflation Reduction Act (IRA), CMS, the federal agency that provides coverage through Medicare, Medicaid, and the Children's Health Insurance Program, was unable to negotiate drug prices for Medicare beneficiaries directly. Instead, this role was assigned to pharmacy benefits managers and insurers tasked with operating the Medicare Part D benefit. Following the passage of the IRA in 2022, CMS is now able to negotiate prices for a small but increasing number of drugs at least 7 years after FDA approval (see Box 5-4).

ALIGNING INNOVATION WITH VALUE

One strategy that is used in other countries to manage drug expenditures is to employ formal value assessments to determine coverage decisions (Mulcahy et al., 2024; Wouters et al., 2025). For instance, in the United Kingdom (UK), the National Institute for Health and Care Excellence (NICE) performs economic evaluations of new drug products, deriving an estimate of cost-effectiveness (Lemley et al., 2020). To determine if the drug is a good value, NICE examines the ratio of cost per quality-adjusted life-year (QALY) gained. If the ratio is under £30,000, NICE is likely to recommend that the National Health Service (NHS) provides coverage for the drug, though considerations for whether the product addresses an unmet

BOX 5-4
Inflation Reduction Act (IRA)

The IRA was enacted in 2022 and is a budget reconciliation bill that adjusted spending for a number of areas, including energy production, clean energy spending, and prescription drug pricing.[a] For the purposes of this box, we will discuss only one of the IRA provisions related to drug pricing that is relevant to this report, although it should be noted that the IRA does a great deal more than what is discussed here.

The IRA put into place a number of policies that, for the first time, allows the government to negotiate prices with manufactures for older brand-name drugs with the highest gross spending in the Medicare program. This Drug Price Negotiation Program requires CMS to directly negotiate with drug manufacturers for up to 20 select drugs that are among the 50 drugs with the highest spending under Medicare Part D (beginning in 2026 with 10 Part D covered drugs) and 50 drugs with the highest spending under Medicare Part B (beginning in 2028 with 20 Part D or Part B covered drugs). CMS can only begin to negotiate prices 7 years after FDA approval for small molecules (with negotiated prices applied 9 years postapproval) and 11 years after FDA approval for biologics (with negotiated prices applied 13 years postapproval). The difference in selection periods between small molecule and biologic drugs was meant to account for the added expense of developing biologics and the existing differences in exclusivity periods granted for these products. However, this provision has been controversial, with many in the pharmaceutical industry arguing that this disincentivizes drug development for small molecules, which some have coined the "pill penalty" (Allen, 2025).

The IRA outlines a number of factors that must be considered when determining the "maximum fair price" for selected drugs to be negotiated (Cubanski, 2025). These include:

1. The R&D costs from manufacturers to develop the drug and the extent to which these costs have been recouped
2. Current production and distribution costs
3. Federal financial support for discovery and development of the drug
4. Comparative effectiveness of the selected drug and its therapeutic alternatives
5. The extent to which the drug and its alternatives address unmet needs for a condition that is not adequately addressed by available therapeutics
6. The extent to which the drug represents a therapeutic advance compared to existing alternatives
7. The comparative effectiveness of the drug and its alternatives.

continued

BOX 5-4 Continued

Therefore, CMS has current authority, although limited to only the drugs under negotiation, to take unmet needs into account when setting drug prices. However, the IRA does not specify how CMS should weigh these different factors when setting drug pricing, and it is unclear the extent to which unmet needs were accounted for in current price negotiations.

The effect that CMS's new authority to negotiate drug prices will have on innovation is not yet clear. Though there is limited anecdotal evidence of individual pharmaceutical companies attributing decisions to cancel investment in individual products to the IRA (Goldman et al., 2023), studies that have modeled the implications of the IRA for future R&D have come to inconsistent conclusions (Vogel et al., 2024b; Xie et al., 2025).

---

^a Inflation Reduction Act of 2022, HR 5376, 117th Congress (2022), https://www.congress.gov/bill/117th-congress/house-bill/5376.

need can be factored into coverage decisions (NICE, 2022). This process ensures that the coverage of a drug product is related to its value, as measured by the additional cost versus the additional health gains. However, NHS has so much negotiating leverage because it is willing to deny access to some drugs for patients if it determines that the value does not justify the price. This can mean that patients do not always have access to drugs they would like, as exemplified a few years ago when a cystic fibrosis drug was not determined to be cost-effective, leaving patients without access (Silverman, 2024). Patients and families fought back, and eventually the manufacturer and NHS reached an agreement (which likely reflects further discounts by the manufacturer, potential increases in the willingness to pay threshold set by NICE, or both). Similarly, economics research has demonstrated that countries with lower expected therapeutic costs tend to have longer delays in access to new therapeutics (Danzon et al., 2005).

Germany, which, like the United States, has a health insurance system with both public and multiple private payers, has its own value assessment program. When a drug comes to market in Germany, manufacturers are guaranteed market access for 1 year at their chosen price (Lemley et al., 2020). During that year, a clinical evaluation of the product is conducted by the German Institute for Quality and Efficiency in Health Care to determine benefit. If the institute determines that there is no added benefit given the availability of other products, the drug's price is based on the lowest price charged within the same drug class. However, if it is determined that the drug does add benefit, negotiations between the regulator and the manufacturer begin, with a completed comparative effectiveness assessment as one factor in these negotiations. Although there are multiple payers in the German system, the negotiations are done at the national level to reduce fragmentation. If negotiations are unsuccessful, then the negotiations enter arbitration and a price is set by a panel. If the manufacturer does not agree with the price, it can opt out of the insurance market or can charge the price of its choosing, with the knowledge that payers will only reimburse patients for the price determined by the panel and that patients will pay the remaining balance if they choose.

Unlike the UK or Germany, the United States has not routinely performed governmental assessments of the value of pharmaceutical products, though this is now a component of the Drug Price Negotiation Program under the IRA. The nonprofit organization Institute for Clinical and Economic Review (ICER) often performs assessments of new drug entrants in the United States, but the resulting estimates are only informative for payers rather than binding (ICER, 2020). Despite the lack of the routine use of such methods, the economic evidence from other resource-high countries suggests that if the United States revised its reimbursement policies by linking pricing to evidence-based value assessments, this could help address areas of misalignment in investments with disease burden and unmet needs by incentivizing industry to invest in the therapeutic areas of highest social value.

Finding 5-14: Many countries negotiate drug prices and set reimbursement terms based on the product's cost-effectiveness, including considerations of unmet need.

CMS already has some limited existing authority to use comparative effectiveness and unmet needs when conducting Medicare price negotiations. As reviewed in Box 5-4, CMS was granted authority through the IRA to include unmet needs and value assessments in price negotiations for the limited number of drugs to be negotiated. However, it is unclear how and if these factors were taken into account in the first round of drugs negotiation. CMS also has existing authority to take comparative effectiveness into account through the New Technology Add-on Payment (NTAP) program.[20]

---

[20] CMS also has similar criteria, including requiring an improvement in clinical outcomes relative to other devices, for pass-through payments for medical devices. However, this criteria does not apply to pass-through payments for drugs, which is the focus of this report, and therefore is not discussed.

NTAP allows for a medical service or technology to receive additional payment beyond the standard Medicare Severity Diagnosis-Related Group (MS-DRG) payment if the new technologies meet three criteria: (1) the medical service or technology must be new; (2) the medical service or technology must be costly such that the MS-DRG rate otherwise applicable to discharges involving the medical service or technology is determined to be inadequate; and (3) the medical service or technology must demonstrate a substantial clinical improvement over existing services or technologies. Therefore, to receive an NTAP designation, CMS is generally, but not always, required to take clinical effectiveness into account, with alternate pathways for NTAP eligibility being developed (CMS, 2024).

These authorities provide some limited negotiating power to CMS to better align pricing with value. However, to more directly tie public insurance prices to unmet need or evidence-supported measures of value, congressional action will be needed to expand the negotiating power that CMS currently has. In taking this action, Congress not only could ensure that pricing matches value, but it could also set terms that maximize patient access, addressing some of the barriers that were discussed in Chapter 4.

> Finding 5-15: CMS has statutory authority to use comparative effectiveness and unmet medical needs for a limited number of older drugs under the Medicare price negotiation and New Technology Add-on Payment (NTAP) programs, but it otherwise lacks authority to control Medicare or Medicaid reimbursement amounts for most new drugs.

> *Conclusion 5-10: If public and private payer reimbursement policies were more aligned with evidence of product value and the extent to which a drug addresses unmet medical need, greater innovation would occur in therapeutic areas with high unmet need.*

> *Conclusion 5-11: Congressional action is needed to more directly tie prices and public insurance reimbursement for novel drugs that address unmet need to evidence-supported measures of value or impact.*

REFERENCES

Abrams, M. T., R. Ramachandran, and R. Steinbrook. 2025. *Report: Failed trials, yet full FDA approval of a Duchenne muscular dystrophy gene therapy.* https://www.citizen.org/article/failed-trials-yet-full-fda-approval-of-a-duchenne-muscular-dystrophy-gene-therapy/ (accessed April 25, 2025).

Acemoglu, D., and J. Linn. 2004. Market size in innovation: Theory and evidence from the pharmaceutical industry. *Quarterly Journal of Economics* 119(3):1049–1090.

Allen, B. 2025. *Three reasons Congress should fix the IRA's pill penalty.* https://phrma.org/blog/congress-needs-to-fix-the-iras-pill-penalty (accessed April 28, 2025).

America's SEED Fund. n.d. *Portfolio.* https://www.sbir.gov/awards (accessed April 17, 2025).

Armstrong, A. 2025a. *Priority review vouchers: By the numbers.* https://www.biospace. com/business/priority-review-vouchers-by-the-numbers#:~:text=FDA%20Priority%20 Review%20Vouchers%20Granted,the%20FDA%20has%20handed%20 out.&text=To%20reflect%20the%20sunsetting%20of,a%20voucher%20from%20 Pharming%20Technologies (accessed April 17, 2025).

Armstrong, A. 2025b. Rare disease biotechs left in a lurch as Congress fails to renew priority review program. *BioSpace,* March 5. https://www.biospace.com/business/rare-disease-biotechs-left-in-a-lurch-as-congress-fails-to-renew-priority-review-program (accessed April 19, 2025).

ARPA-H (Advanced Research Projects Agency for Health). 2024. *About us.* https://arpa-h.gov/ about (accessed March 11, 2025).

Bagley, N., B. Berger, A. Chandra, C. Garthwaite, and A. D. Stern. 2019. The Orphan Drug Act at 35: Observations and an outlook for the twenty-first century. *Innovation Policy and the Economy* 19:97–137.

Barrie, R. 2024. *Switching sales: Investigating the financial impacts of FDA's priority vouchers.* https://www.pharmaceutical-technology.com/features/switching-sales-investigating-the-financial-impacts-of-fdas-priority-vouchers/?cf-view&cf-closed (accessed March 16, 2025).

Beakes-Read, G., M. Neisser, P. Frey, and M. Guarducci. 2022. Analysis of FDA's accelerated approval program performance December 1992–December 2021. *Therapeutic Innovation & Regulatory Science* 56(5):698–703.

Blume-Kohout, M. E., and N. Sood. 2013. Market size and innovation: Effects of Medicare Part D on pharmaceutical research and development. *Journal of Public Economics* 97:327–336.

Bourgeois, F. T., and T. J. Hwang. 2017. The Pediatric Research Equity Act moves into adolescence. *JAMA* 317(3):259–260.

Bourgeois, F. T., and A. S. Kesselheim. 2019. Promoting pediatric drug research and labeling—Outcomes of legislation. *New England Journal of Medicine* 381(9):875–881.

Brennan, Z. 2024. Accelerated approval will be "the norm" for gene therapies, FDA's Peter Marks says. *Endpoints News,* February 27. https://endpts.com/accelerated-approval-will-be-the-norm-for-gene-therapies-fdas-peter-marks-says/ (accessed March 12, 2025).

Buccafusco, C., and J. S. Masur. 2021. Drugs, patents, and well-being. *Washington University Law Review* 98(5):1403–1460.

Budish, E., B. N. Roin, and H. Williams. 2015. Do firms underinvest in long-term research? Evidence from cancer clinical trials. *American Economic Review* 105(7):2044–2085.

Carmack, M., T. Hwang, and F. T. Bourgeois. 2020. Pediatric drug policies supporting safe and effective use of therapeutics in children: A systematic analysis. *Health Affairs* 39(10):1799–1805.

CDC Foundation. 2025. *CDC foundation.* https://www.cdcfoundation.org/ (accessed March 18, 2025).

CMS (Centers for Medicare & Medicaid Services). 2024. *New medical services and new technologies.* https://www.cms.gov/medicare/payment/prospective-payment-systems/acute-inpatient-pps/new-medical-services-and-new-technologies (accessed March 9, 2025).

Congressional Budget Office. 2021. *Research and development in the pharmaceutical industry.* https://www.cbo.gov/publication/57126#_idTextAnchor036 (accessed April 19, 2025).

Congressional Research Service. 2017. *Regulatory exclusivity reform in the 115th Congress.* CRS report R44951. Washington, DC: Congressional Research Service. https://www. congress.gov/crs-product/R44951 (accessed April 19, 2025).

Congressional Research Service. 2022. *Advanced Research Projects Agency for Health (ARPA-H): Congressional action and selected policy issues.* CRS report R47074. Washington, DC: Congressional Research Service. https://www.congress.gov/crs-product/R47074 (accessed April 19, 2025).

Correa-De Araujo, R., W. J. Evans, R. A. Fielding, V. Krishnan, R. H. Carter, J. Appleby, J. Guralnik, L. B. Klickstein, P. Marks, A. A. Moore, S. Peschin, and S. Bhasin. 2023. Synergistic strategies to accelerate the development of function-promoting therapies: Lessons from Operation Warp Speed and oncology drug development. *Journals of Gerontology: Series A* 78(Suppl 1):94–100.

Cubanski, J. 2025. FAQ about the Inflation Reduction Act's Medicare drug price negotiation program. *KFF*, January 23. https://www.kff.org/medicare/issue-brief/faqs-about-the-inflation-reduction-acts-medicare-drug-price-negotiation-program/#negotiating-factors (accessed March 8, 2025).

Cubanski, J., M. Rae, K. Young, and A. Damico. 2019. How does prescription drug spending and use compare across large employer plans, Medicare Part D, and Medicaid? *KFF*, May 20. https://www.kff.org/medicare/issue-brief/how-does-prescription-drug-spending-and-use-compare-across-large-employer-plans-medicare-part-d-and-medicaid/ (accessed January 2, 2025).

Cudkowicz, M., M. K. Chase, C. S. Coffey, D. J. Ecklund, B. J. Thornell, C. Lungu, K. Mahoney, L. Gutmann, J. M. Shefner, K. J. Staley, M. Bosch, E. Foster, J. D. Long, E. O. Bayman, J. Torner, J. Yankey, R. Peters, T. Huff, R. A. Conwit, NeuroNEXT Clinical Study Sites, et al. 2020. Seven-year experience from the National Institute of Neurological Disorders and Stroke–supported network for excellence in neuroscience clinical trials. *JAMA Neurology* 77(6):755–763.

Daniel, M. G., T. M. Pawlik, A. N. Fader, N. F. Esnaola, and M. A. Makary. 2016. The Orphan Drug Act: Restoring the mission to rare diseases. *American Journal of Clinical Oncology* 39(2):210–213.

Danzon, P. M., Y. R. Wang, and L. Wang. 2005. The impact of price regulation on the launch delay of new drugs—Evidence from twenty-five major markets in the 1990s. *Health Economics* 14(3):269–292.

Darrow, J. J., J. Avorn, and A. S. Kesselheim. 2018. The FDA breakthrough-drug designation—Four years of experience. *New England Journal of Medicine* 378(15):1444–1453.

Department of Commerce. 2021. *USPTO has opportunities to improve its internal controls and oversight related to PTA and PTE calculations.* U.S. Department of Commerce.

D'Souza, A., K. Hoyt, C. Snyder, and A. Stapp. 2024. *Can Operation Warp Speed serve as a model for accelerating innovations beyond COVID vaccines?* National Bureau of Economic Research working paper 32831. https://www.nber.org/papers/w32831 (accessed April 20, 2025).

Dolgin, E. 2019. Massive NIH–industry project opens portals to target validation. *Nature Reviews Drug Discovery* 18(4):240–242.

Downing, N. S., N. D. Shah, J. A. Aminawung, A. M. Pease, J. D. Zeitoun, H. M. Krumholz, and J. S. Ross. 2017. Postmarket safety events among novel therapeutics approved by the U.S. Food and Drug Administration between 2001 and 2010. *JAMA* 317(18):1854–1863.

Dranove, D., C. Garthwaite, and M. Hermosilla. 2020. *Expected profits and the scientific novelty of innovation.* National Bureau of Economic Research working paper 27093. https://www.nber.org/papers/w27093 (accessed April 20, 2025).

Dubois, P., O. De Mouzon, F. Scott-Morton, and P. Seabright. 2015. Market size and pharmaceutical innovation. *RAND Journal of Economics* 46(4):844–871.

Duggan, M., and F. M. Scott Morton. 2006. The distortionary effects of government procurement: Evidence from Medicaid prescription drug purchasing. *Quarterly Journal of Economics* 121(1):1–30.

Dutta, S., J. Rodrigues, and T. B. Folta. 2023. Does NIH select the right healthcare ventures through the SBIR grant program? *Journal of Technology Transfer* 48(4):1206–1220.

Dyachkova, Y., C. Dunger-Baldauf, N. Barbier, J. Devenport, S. Franzén, G. Kazeem, T. Künzel, P. Mancini, G. Mordenti, K. Richert, A. Ridolfi, and D. Saure. 2024. Do you want to stay single? Considerations on single-arm trials in drug development and the postregulatory space. *Pharmaceutical Statistics* 23(6):1206–1217.

Eglovitch, J. S. 2024. Convergence: FDA officials offer updates on START, STAR pilots. *Regulatory Focus*, September 24. https://www.raps.org/news-and-articles/news-articles/2024/9/convergence-fda-officials-offer-updates-on-start, (accessed April 19, 2025).

Eisenberg, R. S. 2007. The role of the FDA in innovation policy. *Michigan Telecommunications & Technology Law Review* 13(2):345–388.

Eisenberg, P., P. Kaufmann, E. Sigal, and J. Woodcock. 2012. Appendix G: Discussion Paper: Developing a Clinical Trials Infrastructure, in *Envisioning a Transformed Clinical Trials Enterprise in the United States: Establishing an Agenda for 2020: Workshop Summary*. Washington, DC: The National Academies Press.

EPA (Environmental Protection Agency). 2024. *Frequently asked questions about the Federal Technology Transfer Act program.* https://www.epa.gov/ftta/frequently-asked-questions-about-federal-technology-transfer-act-program#:~:text=If%20the%20invention%20occurred%20under%20a%20CRADA%2C,for%20an%20exclusive%20license%20on%20the%20technology (accessed April 27, 2025).

Fashoyin-Aje, L. A., G. U. Mehta, J. A. Beaver, and R. Pazdur. 2022. The on- and off-ramps of oncology accelerated approval. *New England Journal of Medicine* 387(16):1439–1442.

FDA (Food and Drug Administration). n.d. *Exclusivity and generic drugs: What does it mean?* https://www.fda.gov/files/drugs/published/Exclusivity-and-Generic-Drugs--What-Does-It-Mean-.pdf (accessed June 1, 2025).

FDA. 2005. *Guidance for industry: How to comply with the Pediatric Research Equity Act.* Rockville, MD: Center for Drug Evaluation and Research, Food and Drug Administration. https://www.fda.gov/media/72274/download (accessed April 19, 2025).

FDA. 2017. *FDA drug competition action plan.* https://www.fda.gov/drugs/guidance-compliance-regulatory-information/fda-drug-competition-action-plan (accessed April 2, 2025).

FDA. 2018a. *Breakthrough therapy.* https://www.fda.gov/patients/fast-track-breakthrough-therapy-accelerated-approval-priority-review/breakthrough-therapy (accessed January 4, 2025).

FDA. 2018b. *Priority review.* https://www.fda.gov/patients/fast-track-breakthrough-therapy-accelerated-approval-priority-review/priority-review (accessed March 12, 2025).

FDA. 2021. *Accelerating Access to Critical Therapies for ALS Act – ACT for ALS.* https://www.fda.gov/industry/medical-products-rare-diseases-and-conditions/accelerating-access-critical-therapies-als-act-act-als (accessed March 11, 2025).

FDA. 2022a. *Action plan for rare neurodegenerative diseases including amyotrophic lateral sclerosis.* Rockville, MD: Center for Drug Evaluation and Research, Food and Drug Administration. https://www.fda.gov/media/159372/download (accessed April 19, 2025).

FDA. 2022b. *Rare Disease Endpoint Advancement pilot program.* https://www.fda.gov/drugs/development-resources/rare-disease-endpoint-advancement-pilot-program (accessed April 11, 2025).

FDA. 2023. *Split Real-Time Application Review (STAR).* https://www.fda.gov/drugs/development-resources/split-real-time-application-review-star (accessed March 12, 2025).

FDA. 2024a. *Accelerating Rare Disease Cures (ARC) year two: Annual report driving innovation through scientific and regulatory advancement.* Silver Spring, MD: Center for Drug Evaluation and Research, Food and Drug Administration. https://www.fda.gov/media/182662/download (accessed April 19, 2025).

FDA. 2024b. *Breakthrough therapy.* https://www.fda.gov/patients/fast-track-breakthrough-therapy-accelerated-approval-priority-review/breakthrough-therapy (accessed April 11, 2025).

FDA. 2024c. *Designating an orphan product: Drugs and biological products.* https://www.fda. gov/industry/medical-products-rare-diseases-and-conditions/designating-orphan-product-drugs-and-biological-products (accessed April 17, 2025).

FDA. 2024d. *Fast track.* https://www.fda.gov/patients/fast-track-breakthrough-therapy-accelerated-approval-priority-review/fast-track (accessed January 26, 2025).

FDA. 2024e. *Fast track, breakthrough therapy, accelerated approval, priority review.* https://www.fda.gov/patients/learn-about-drug-and-device-approvals/fast-track-breakthrough-therapy-accelerated-approval-priority-review (accessed April 11, 2025).

FDA. 2024f. *FDA Rare Disease Innovation Hub to enhance and advance outcomes for patients.* https://www.fda.gov/news-events/fda-voices/fda-rare-disease-innovation-hub-enhance-and-advance-outcomes-patients (accessed April 11, 2025).

FDA. 2024g. *LEADER 3D: Learning and Education to Advance and Empower Rare Disease Drug Developers.* https://www.fda.gov/about-fda/accelerating-rare-disease-cures-arc-program/learning-and-education-advance-and-empower-rare-disease-drug-developers-leader-3d (accessed June 1, 2025).

FDA. 2024h. *Platform technology designation program for drug development: Guidance for industry.* Rockville, MD: Food and Drug Administration. https://www.fda.gov/media/178938/download (accessed April 20, 2025).

FDA. 2024i. *Rare pediatric disease designation and priority review voucher programs.* https://www.fda.gov/industry/medical-products-rare-diseases-and-conditions/rare-pediatric-disease-designation-and-priority-review-voucher-programs (accessed January 27, 2025).

FDA 2024j. *Real-Time Oncology Review.* https://www.fda.gov/about-fda/oncology-center-excellence/real-time-oncology-review (accessed March 12, 2025).

FDA. 2024k. *Support for Clinical Trials Advancing Rare Disease Therapeutics (START) pilot program.* https://www.fda.gov/science-research/clinical-trials-and-human-subject-protection/support-clinical-trials-advancing-rare-disease-therapeutics-start-pilot-program (accessed March 12, 2025).

FDA. 2025a. *Accelerated approval and considerations for determining whether a confirmatory trial is underway.* Silver Spring, MD: Food and Drug Administration. https://www.fda.gov/media/184831/download (accessed April 20, 2025).

FDA. 2025b. *Advancing health through innovation: New drug therapy approvals 2024.* https://www.fda.gov/drugs/novel-drug-approvals-fda/novel-drug-approvals-2024 (accessed May 15, 2025).

FDA. 2025c. *FDA Rare Disease Innovation Hub.* https://www.fda.gov/industry/medical-products-rare-diseases-and-conditions/fda-rare-disease-innovation-hub (accessed March 12, 2025).

FDA. 2025d. *Learning and Education to Advance and Empower Rare Disease Drug Developers (LEADER 3D).* https://www.fda.gov/about-fda/accelerating-rare-disease-cures-arc-program/learning-and-education-advance-and-empower-rare-disease-drug-developers-leader-3d (accessed March 11, 2025).

FDA. 2025e. *Rare Disease Innovation Hub strategic agenda 2025.* Silver Spring, MD: Center for Drug Evaluation and Research. https://www.fda.gov/media/185144/download (accessed April 19, 2025).

FDA. 2025f. *21st Century Cures Act: MCM-related cures provisions.* https://www.fda.gov/emergency-preparedness-and-response/mcm-legal-regulatory-and-policy-framework/21st-century-cures-act-mcm-related-cures-provisions (accessed May 16, 2025).

Fernandez Lynch, H. 2023. *Hearing on "Unlocking hope: Access to therapies for people with rare, progressive, and serious diseases."* U.S. Congress, Senate, Subcommittee on Aging. https://www.aging.senate.gov/imo/media/doc/a5bc7959-d2b7-8abf-400b-f3cd46744c8a/Testimony_Fernandez%20Lynch%2010.26.23.pdf (accessed June 4, 2025).

Fernandez Lynch, H., and A. Bateman-House. 2020. Facilitating both evidence and access: Improving FDA's accelerated approval and expanded access pathways. *Journal of Law, Medicine & Ethics* 48(2):365–372.

Fernandez Lynch, H., R. E. Sachs, S. Lee, M. Herder, J. S. Ross, and R. Ramachandran. 2023. Extending the U.S. Food and Drug Administration's postmarket authorities. *JAMA Health Forum* 4(6):e231313.

Feuerstein, A., and D. Garde. 2024. Amylyx ALS drug failure leaves patients, advocates, and researchers reeling — and wondering what's next. *STAT News*. https://www.statnews.com/2024/03/08/amylyx-pharmaceuticals-als-amyotrophic-lateral-sclerosis-drug-rely-vrio-failure/ (accessed April 25, 2025).

Finkelstein, A. 2004. Static and dynamic effects of health policy: Evidence from the vaccine industry. *Quarterly Journal of Economics* 119(2):527–564.

Floersh, H. 2024. *Denali, Neurogene and more picked by FDA's 'Operation Warp Speed' for rare disease*. https://www.fiercebiotech.com/research/fda-selects-denali-neurogene-larimar-and-grace-sciences-rare-disease-therapy-pilot (accessed March 12, 2025).

FNIH (Foundation for the National Institutes of Health). 2024. *AMP Symposium Day 1: Panel Discussion - 10 Years of AMP Impacts*, February 28. https://www.youtube.com/watch?v=ZfySJxtdXdg (accessed May 16, 2025).

FNIH. 2025a. *AMP Bespoke Gene Therapy Consortium (BGTC)*. https://fnih.org/our-programs/accelerating-medicines-partnership-amp/bespoke-gene-therapy-consortium-bgtc/ (accessed March 17, 2025).

FNIH. 2025b. *FNIH*. https://fnih.org/ (accessed March 18, 2025).

FNIH. 2025c. *Ultra-rare cancer treatment advancement program design phase*. https://fnih.org/our-programs/ultra-rare-cancer-treatment-advancement/ (accessed July 25, 2025).

Galkina Cleary, E., M. J. Jackson, E. W. Zhou, and F. D. Ledley. 2023. Comparison of research spending on new drug approvals by the National Institutes of Health vs the pharmaceutical industry, 2010-2019. *JAMA Health Forum* 4(4):e230511.

Gallo, M. E., and H. B. Hogue. 2022. *Agency-related nonprofit research foundations and corporations*. CRS report R46109. Washington, DC: Congressional Research Service. https://www.congress.gov/crs-product/R46109 (accessed April 20, 2025).

GAO (Government Accountability Office). 2020. *Drug development: FDA's priority review voucher programs*. GAO-20-251. Washington, DC: Government Accountability Office. https://www.gao.gov/products/gao-20-251 (accessed April 19, 2025).

GHIT Fund (Global Health Innovative Technology Fund). 2025. *Fight neglected diseases through partnerships*. https://www.ghitfund.org/ (accessed April 20, 2025).

Giaccotto, C., E. Rexford, E. Santerre, and J. A. Vernon. 2005. Drug prices and research and development investment behavior in the pharmaceutical industry. *Journal of Law and Economics* 48(1):195–214.

Goldman, M. 2012. The Innovative Medicines Initiative: A European response to the innovation challenge. *Clinical Pharmacology & Therapeutics* 91(3):418–425.

Goldman, M., A. Wittelsberger, and M. T. De Magistris. 2013. The Innovative Medicines Initiative moves translational immunology forward. *European Journal of Immunology* 43(2):298–302.

Goldman, D., J. Grogan, D. Lakdawalla, B. Liden, J. Shafrin, K.-S. Than, and E. Trish. 2023. *Mitigating the Inflation Reduction Act's adverse impacts on the prescription drug market*. USC Leonard D. Schaeffer Center for Health Policy & Economics. https://schaeffer.usc.edu/wp-content/uploads/2024/10/2023.04_Schaeffer-White-Paper_Mitigating-Adverse-Impacts-of-the-IRA.pdf (accessed May 16, 2025).

Grabowski, H., and J. Vernon. 2000. The determinants of pharmaceutical research and development expenditures. *Journal of Evolutionary Economics* 10(1–2):201–215.

Greenberg, K. S., H. F. Lynch, C. Nwakama, J. Frumovitz, S. Setru, A. M. Johnson, S. M. Shah, L. Schadt, M. S. McCoy, A. K. Hoffman, and E. A. Largent. 2025. A review of public comments submitted to the Centers for Medicare and Medicaid Services in response to the 2022 national coverage decision on treatment for Alzheimer's disease. *Journal of Law and the Biosciences* 12(1).

Greene, J. A., and S. H. Podolsky. 2012. Reform, regulation, and pharmaceuticals — the Kefauver–Harris amendments at 50. *New England Journal of Medicine* 367(16):1481–1483.

Gyawali, B., S. P. Hey, and A. S. Kesselheim. 2019. Assessment of the clinical benefit of cancer drugs receiving accelerated approval. *JAMA Internal Medicine* 179(7):906–913.

HHS (U.S. Department of Health and Human Services). 2018. *2018 NCI overview: Economic impact analysis of the NCI SBIR program.* https://sbir.cancer.gov/portfolio/impact-study/economic-impact-study-summary.pdf (accessed April 19, 2025).

HHS. 2023. *Real-Time Oncology Review (RTOR) guidance for industry.* https://www.fda.gov/media/173641/download (accessed June 1, 2025).

HHS. 2025. *How FDA used its accelerated approval pathway raised concerns in 3 of 24 drugs reviewed.* Washington, DC: Department of Health and Human Services, Office of the Inspector General. https://oig.hhs.gov/reports/all/2025/how-fda-used-its-accelerated-approval-pathway-raised-concerns-in-3-of-24-drugs-reviewed (accessed April 20, 2025).

Hoffmann, D., S. Van Dalsem, and F. S. David. 2019. Stock price effects of breakthrough therapy designation. *Nature Reviews Drug Discovery* 18(3):165.

Homeland Security Science and Technology. 2020. *CRADA fact sheet.* https://www.dhs.gov/publication/crada-factsheet (accessed April 20, 2025).

Howell, S. T. 2017. Financing innovation: Evidence from R&D grants. *American Economic Review* 107(4):1136–1164.

Hwang, T. J., F. T. Bourgeois, J. M. Franklin, and A. S. Kesselheim. 2019a. Impact of the priority review voucher program on drug development for rare pediatric diseases. *Health Affairs (Millwood)* 38(2):313–319.

Hwang, T. J., L. Orenstein, A. S. Kesselheim, and F. T. Bourgeois. 2019b. Completion rate and reporting of mandatory pediatric postmarketing studies under the U.S. Pediatric Research Equity Act. *JAMA Pediatrics* 173(1):68–74.

ICER (Institute for Clinical and Economic Review). 2020. *2020-2023 value assessment framework.* https://icer.org/wp-content/uploads/2020/10/ICER_2020_2023_VAF_102220.pdf (accessed June 1, 2025).

IOM (Institute of Medicine). 1998. *Scientific opportunities and public needs: Improving priority setting and public input at the National Institutes of Health.* Washington, DC: National Academy Press.

IOM. 2010. *Rare diseases and orphan products: Accelerating research and development.* Washington, DC: The National Academies Press.

IOM. 2012. *Envisioning a transformed clinical trials enterprise in the United States: Establishing an agenda for 2020: Workshop summary.* Washington, DC: The National Academies Press.

IQVIA. 2019. *Global approaches to drug development: When ex-US clinical data can support US drug approvals.* https://www.iqvia.com/-/media/iqvia/pdfs/library/white-papers/global-approaches-to-drug-development.pdf (accessed June 1, 2025).

Jackson Foundation (Henry M. Jackson Foundation for the Advancement of Military Medicine). 2025. *Who we are.* https://www.hjf.org/about-hjf (accessed March 18, 2025).

Jain, N., T. Hwang, J. M. Franklin, and A. S. Kesselheim. 2017. Association of the priority review voucher with neglected tropical disease drug and vaccine development. JAMA 318(4):388.

Johnston, J. L., J. S. Ross, and R. Ramachandran. 2023. U.S. Food and Drug Administration approval of drugs not meeting pivotal trial primary end points, 2018–2021. *JAMA Internal Medicine* 183(4):376.

Joseph, A. 2024. Dispute over Duchenne gene therapy highlights thorny access issues. *STAT News*, September 27. https://www.statnews.com/2024/09/27/duchenne-muscular-dystrophy-sarepta-elevidys-insurance-issues/ (accessed March 21, 2025).

Kapczynski, A. 2018. Dangerous times: The FDA's role in information production, past and future. *Minnesota Law Review* 102:2357–2382.

Kaplan, R. M., A. J. Koong, and V. Irvin. 2023. Review of evidence supporting 2022 U.S. Food and Drug Administration drug approvals. *JAMA Network Open* 6(8):e2327650.

Keisler-Starkey, K., and L. N. Bunch. 2024. *Health insurance coverage in the United States: 2023.* U.S. Census Bureau report no. p60-284. https://www.census.gov/library/publications/2024/demo/p60-284.html (accessed April 20, 2025).

Keshtkar-Jahromi, M., K. J. Anstrom, C. Barkauskas, S. M. Brown, E. S. Daar, W. Fischer, K. W. Gibbs, E. S. Higgs, M. D. Hughes, P. Jagannathan, L. Lavange, C. J. Lindsell, S. U. Nayak, R. Paredes, M. Parmar, I. D. Peltan, M. Proschan, M. S. Shotwell, D. M. Vock, T. Yokum, and S. J. Adam. 2024. ACTIV trials: Lessons learned in trial design in the setting of an emergent pandemic. *Journal of Clinical and Translational Science* 8(1).

Kesselheim, A. S. 2020. *Congress should support development of new treatments for pediatric rare diseases, but not with priority review vouchers.* https://docs.house.gov/meetings/IF/IF14/20200729/110949/HMTG-116-IF14-Wstate-KesselheimA-20200729.pdf (accessed June 1, 2025).

Lakdawalla, D. N., and N. Sood. 2012. 143 incentives to innovate. In P. M. Danzon and S. Nicholson (eds.), *The Oxford handbook of the economics of the biopharmaceutical industry.* New York: Oxford University Press. Pp. 143–166.

Lalani, H. S., S. Nagar, A. Sarpatwari, R. E. Barenie, J. Avorn, B. N. Rome, and A. S. Kesselheim. 2023. U.S. public investment in development of mRNA COVID-19 vaccines: Retrospective cohort study. *BMJ* 380:e073747.

Ledley, F. D., and E. Galkina Cleary. 2023. NIH funding for patents that contribute to market exclusivity of drugs approved 2010-2019 and the public interest protections of Bayh-Dole. *PLOS One* 18(7):e0288447.

Lee, D., E. Stein, and N. Gooneratne. 2021. *SBIR/STTR grants: Introduction and overview.* Academic Entrepreneurship for Medical and Health Sciences. https://academicentrepreneurship.pubpub.org/pub/1elox915/release/5 (accessed July 17, 2025).

Lemley, M. A., L. L. Ouellette, and R. E. Sachs. 2020. The Medicare innovation subsidy. *New York University Law Review* 95(1):95–96.

Liang, W. 2024. Support for clinical Trials Advancing Rare disease Therapeutics (START) pilot. https://www.fda.gov/media/176596/download (accessed June 1, 2025).

Lietzan, E., and K. M. Lybecker. 2020. Distorted drug patents. *Washington Law Review* 95(3):1317–1381.

Liu, I. T. T., and A. S. Kesselheim. 2024. Clinical benefit and revenues of drugs affected by rare pediatric disease priority review vouchers, 2017-2023. *Journal of Pediatrics* 275.

Liu, I. T. T., A. S. Kesselheim, and E. R. S. Cliff. 2024. Clinical benefit and regulatory outcomes of cancer drugs receiving accelerated approval. *JAMA* 331(17):1471–1479.

Meadows, M. 2006. Promoting safe & effective drugs for 100 years. *FDA Consumer Magazine*, February.

MedPAC (Medicare Payment Advisory Commission). 2023. Addressing high prices of drugs covered under Medicare Part B. Chapter 1 in Medicare Payment Advisory Commission, *Report to the Congress: Medicare and the health care delivery system.* Washington, DC: MedPAC. Pp. 3–66.

Menetski, J. P., S. C. Hoffmann, S. S. Cush, T. N. Kamphaus, C. P. Austin, P. L. Herrling, and J. A. Wagner. 2019. The Foundation for the National Institutes of Health Biomarkers Consortium: Past accomplishments and new strategic direction. *Clinical Pharmacology & Therapeutics* 105(4):829–843.

Miller, K. L., A. D. Stern, A. Kearsley, and J. Kao. 2024. FDA breakthrough therapy designation reduced late-stage drug development time. *Health Affairs* 43(7):1003–1010.

Mooghali, M., A. Mohammad, J. D. Wallach, A. P. Mitchell, J. S. Ross, and R. Ramachandran. 2024a. Premarket evidence and postmarketing requirements for Real-Time Oncology Review indication approvals. *JAMA Network Open* 7(5):e249233.

Mooghali, M., J. D. Wallach, J. S. Ross, and R. Ramachandran. 2024b. Premarket pivotal trial end points and postmarketing requirements for FDA breakthrough therapies. *JAMA Network Open* 7(8):e2430486.

Mulcahy, A. W., D. Schwam, and S. L. Lovejoy. 2024. *International prescription drug price comparisons: Estimates using 2022 data.* Santa Monica, CA: RAND Corporation. https://www.rand.org/pubs/periodicals/health-quarterly/issues/v11/n3/05.html (accessed April 20, 2025).

NASEM (National Academies of Sciences, Engineering, and Medicine). 2015. *SBIR/STTR at the National Institutes of Health.* Washington, DC: The National Academies Press.

NASEM. 2022a. *Assessment of the SBIR and STTR programs at the National Institutes of Health.* Washington, DC: The National Academies Press.

NASEM. 2022b. *Envisioning a transformed clinical trials enterprise for 2030: Proceedings of a workshop.* Washington, DC: The National Academies Press.

NASEM. 2023a. *Review of the SBIR and STTR programs at the National Science Foundation.* Washington, DC: The National Academies Press.

NASEM. 2023b. *The Food and Drug Administration's accelerated approval process for new pharmaceuticals: Proceedings of a workshop—in brief.* Washington, DC: The National Academies Press.

NASEM. 2024a. *Advancing clinical research with pregnant and lactating populations: Overcoming real and perceived liability risks.* Washington, DC: The National Academies Press.

NASEM. 2024b. *Preventing and treating dementia: Research priorities to accelerate progress.* Washington, DC: The National Academies Press.

NASEM. 2024c. *Regulatory processes for rare disease drugs in the United States and European Union: Flexibilities and collaborative opportunities.* Washington, DC: The National Academies Press.

Naval Postgraduate School. 2022. *CRADA 101.* https://nps.edu/documents/103449465/0/How%2Bto%2Bwork%2Bwith%2BNPS_CRADA.pdf (accessed April 20, 2025).

NCATS (National Center for Advancing Translational Sciences). 2021. *NIH, FDA and 15 private organizations join forces to increase effective gene therapies for rare diseases.* https://ncats.nih.gov/news-events/news/2021/nih-fda-and-15-private-organizations-join-forces-to-increase-effective-gene-therapies-for-rare-diseases (accessed April 28, 2025).

NCATS. 2024. *BrIDG.* https://ncats.nih.gov/research/research-activities/bridgs (accessed March 14, 2025).

NCI (National Cancer Institute). n.d.-a. NCI experimental therapeutics program (NExT): A government, academic, industry partnership for cancer drug discovery/development. https://rrp.cancer.gov/working_groups/20230705_NExT_Program_Slide_Deck.pdf (accessed June 1, 2025).

NCI. n.d.-b. *NExT NCI experimental therapeutics program.* https://next.cancer.gov/ (accessed March 14, 2025).

NeuroNEXT. n.d. *Network for excellence in neuroscience clinical trials.* https://neuronext.org/ (accessed March 13, 2025).

NICE (National Institute for Health and Care Excellence). 2022. *NICE health technology evaluations: The manual.* https://www.nice.org.uk/process/pmg36/resources/nice-health-technology-evaluations-the-manual-pdf-72286779244741 (accessed May 16, 2025).

NIH (National Institutes of Health). 2020. *NIH launches clinical trials network to test COVID-19 vaccines and other prevention tools.* https://www.nih.gov/news-events/news-releases/nih-launches-clinical-trials-network-test-covid-19-vaccines-other-prevention-tools (accessed March 11, 2025).

NIH. 2024a. *NIH to award over $207 million to support highly innovative biomedical and behavioral research projects.* https://commonfund.nih.gov/highrisk/news/nih-award-over-207-million-support-highly-innovative-biomedical-and-behavioral (accessed February 28, 2025).

NIH. 2024b. *Simplified peer review framework.* https://grants.nih.gov/policy-and-compliance/policy-topics/peer-review/simplifying-review/framework (accessed March 14, 2025).

NIH Common Fund. 2025. *Welcome to the NIH Common Fund.* https://commonfund.nih.gov/ (accessed April 16, 2025).

NIH Office of Technology Transfer. n.d. *CRADAs.* https://www.techtransfer.nih.gov/partnerships/cradas (accessed March 14, 2025).

NIH SEED. n.d. *Understanding SBIR and STTR.* https://seed.nih.gov/small-business-funding/small-business-program-basics/understanding-sbir-sttr#Budget-and-timelines-for-funding (accessed April 17, 2025).

NINDS (National Institute of Neurological Disorders and Stroke). 2025. *NeuroNEXT: Network for excellence in neuroscience clinical trials.* https://www.ninds.nih.gov/current-research/research-funded-ninds/clinical-research/neuronext-network-excellence-neuroscience-clinical-trials (accessed April 27, 2025).

Olson, M. K., and N. Yin. 2018. Examining firm responses to R&D policy: An analysis of pediatric exclusivity. *American Journal of Health Economics* 4(3):321–357.

Parasrampuria, S. and S. Murphy. 2024. *Comparing U.S. and international market size and average pricing for prescription drugs, 2017–2022.* Washington, DC: Office of the Assistant Secretary for Planning and Evaluation, U.S. Department of Health and Human Services. https://aspe.hhs.gov/sites/default/files/documents/4326cc7fe43bc11770598cf2a13f478c/international-market-size-prices.pdf (accessed April 20, 2025).

Pharmaceutical Law Group. 2021. *The enduring role of orphan drug exclusivity for biologics.* https://www.pharmalawgrp.com/blog/13/the-enduring-role-of-orphan-drug-exclusivity-for-biologics/#:~:text=Many%20new%20biologics%20receive%20Orphan,common%20date%20of%20drug%20approval (accessed April 17, 2025).

Pierson, L., and J. Millum. 2022. Health research priority setting: Do grant review processes reflect ethical principles? *Global Public Health* 17(7):1186–1199.

Piller, C. 2022. Blots on a field? *Science* 377(6604):358–363. https://www.science.org/content/article/potential-fabrication-research-images-threatens-key-theory-alzheimers-disease (accessed March 17, 2025).

Reagan-Udall Foundation for the FDA. 2022. *COVID-19 lessons learned: Clinical evaluation of therapeutics—Workshop summary.* Washington, DC: Reagan-Udall Foundation for the FDA. https://reaganudall.org/sites/default/files/2022-07/062822_COVID%20Response_Final_CORRECTED.pdf (accessed April 20, 2025).

Ridley, D. B. 2017. Priorities for the priority review voucher. *American Society of Tropical Medicine and Hygiene* 96(1):14–15.

Ridley, D. B., and S. A. Régnier. 2016. The commercial market for priority review vouchers. *Health Affairs* 35(5):776–783.

Rome, B. N., A. C. Egilman, and A. S. Kesselheim. 2022. Trends in prescription drug launch prices, 2008-2021. *JAMA* 327(21):2145.

Romond, E. H., E. A. Perez, J. Bryant, V. J. Suman, C. E. Geyer, N. E. Davidson, E. Tan-Chiu, S. Martino, S. Paik, P. A. Kaufman, S. M. Swain, T. M. Pisansky, L. Fehrenbacher, L. A. Kutteh, V. G. Vogel, D. W. Visscher, G. Yothers, R. B. Jenkins, A. M. Brown, S. R. Dakhil, E. P. Mamounas, W. L. Lingle, P. M. Klein, J. N. Ingle, and N. Wolmark. 2005. Trastuzumab plus adjuvant chemotherapy for operable HER2-positive breast cancer. *New England Journal of Medicine* 353(16):1673-1684.

Sampat, B., P. Azoulay, P. Stephan, C. Franzoni, L. L. Ouellette, K. Myers, M. Durvasula, R. Cook-Deegan, and R. Holt. 2023. *Building a better NIH.* [Collection of papers.] https://www.brookings.edu/collection/building-a-better-nih/ (accessed April 19, 2025).

Sarpatwari, A., R. F. Beall, A. Abdurrob, M. He, and A. S. Kesselheim. 2018. Evaluating the impact of the Orphan Drug Act's seven-year market exclusivity period. *Health Affairs* 37(5):732–737.

SBA (Small Business Administration). 2025. *Agency resources.* https://www.americasseedfund.us/resources (accessed March 11, 2025).

SEED. n.d. *Navigate NIH's research areas.* https://seed.nih.gov/small-business-funding/funding-by-research-area (accessed March 13, 2025).

Silverman, E. 2024. Vertex reaches a new deal with NHS England over its pricey cystic fibrosis treatments. *STAT News,* June 20. https://www.statnews.com/pharmalot/2024/06/20/vertex-uk-england-nhs-cystic-fibrosis-trikafta-medicines/ (accessed March 9, 2025).

Sinha, M. S., A. D. Stern, and A. K. Rai. 2024. Four decades of orphan drugs and priorities for the future. *New England Journal of Medicine* 391(2):100–102.

Sorkin, A. 2023. HHS SBIR contract RFP informational webinar. NIH SEED. https://seed.nih.gov/sites/default/files/2023-10/SBIR-Contracts-PHS-2024-1-Slides.pdf (accessed June 1, 2025).

STIP (Department of Energy Scientific and Technical Information Program). n.d. *CRADA: References and key excerpts.* https://www.osti.gov/stip/submit/submission-basics/protected-sti/crada (accessed April 27, 2025).

Sukhatme, N. U., and M. G. Bloche. 2019. Health care costs and the arc of innovation. *Minnesota Law Review* 104(2):955–1040.

Thomas, S., and A. Caplan. 2019. The Orphan Drug Act revisited. *JAMA* 321(9):833–834.

Vereshchagina, L. 2022. *Three things to know about the accelerated approval pathway.* PhRMA. https://phrma.org/blog/three-things-to-know-about-the-accelerated-approval-pathway (accessed May 23, 2025).

Vernon, J. A. 2005. Examining the link between price regulation and pharmaceutical R&D investment. *Health Economics* 14(1):1–16.

Vogel, M., O. Zhao, W. B. Feldman, A. Chandra, A. S. Kesselheim, and B. N. Rome. 2024a. Cost of exempting sole orphan drugs from Medicare negotiation. *JAMA Internal Medicine* 184(1):63–69.

Vogel, M., P. Kakani, A. Chandra, and R. M. Conti. 2024b. Medicare price negotiation and pharmaceutical innovation following the Inflation Reduction Act. *Nature Biotechnology* 42(3):406–412.

Wong, A. K., M. Mooghali, R. Ramachandran, J. S. Ross, and J. D. Wallach. 2023. Use of expedited regulatory programs and clinical development times for FDA-approved novel therapeutics. *JAMA Network Open* 6(8):e2331753.

Wouters, O. J., S. D. Sullivan, E. M. Cousin, N. Gabriel, I. Papanicolas, and I. Hernandez. 2025. Drug prices negotiated by Medicare vs U.S. net prices and prices in other countries. *JAMA* 333(1):85–87.

Xie, R. Z., T. Cameron, and P. Kolchinsky. 2025. The impact of the Inflation Reduction Act on investment in innovative medicines: A project-level analysis. *Therapeutic Innovation & Regulatory Science* 59(3):409–417.

Yin, W. 2008. Market incentives and pharmaceutical innovation. *Journal of Health Economics* 27(4):1060–1077.

Zhang, A. D., J. Puthumana, N. S. Downing, N. D. Shah, H. M. Krumholz, and J. S. Ross. 2020. Assessment of clinical trials supporting U.S. Food and Drug Administration approval of novel therapeutic agents, 1995-2017. *JAMA Network Open* 3(4):e203284

6

Recommendations

Therapeutic innovation in the United States has powered medical innovation around the world, but despite significant public and private investment, unmet medical needs remain. To better understand what drives mismatches among investment, disease burden, and unmet need and to inform their deliberations, the committee gathered and synthesized information from the literature and public testimony. This information is summarized in the preceding chapters, which analyze patterns of mismatch among investment, burden, and unmet need (Chapter 3); explore reasons driving this mismatch (Chapter 4); and discuss policy strategies to improve alignment (Chapter 5). Figure 6-1 outlines the committee's conceptual approach to their charge, including identifying misalignments and the barriers to achieving alignment, employing levers of change to address misalignments, and the intermediate- and long-term outcomes that can be achieved.

This chapter presents the committee's specific recommendations to better align investments in therapeutic development with disease burden and unmet need. Recognizing the complex, multisector landscape of therapeutic development, the committee identified several key areas for strategic action: public health data collation and availability, public investment in biomedical research, public–private partnerships, the regulatory environment, and payment and reimbursement policy incentives. The committee's recommendations are thus organized around five goals:

1. Design a state-of-the-art publicly accessible system to assess and track unmet need associated with U.S. disease burden, with a critical focus on identifying areas of mismatch and reducing health disparities.

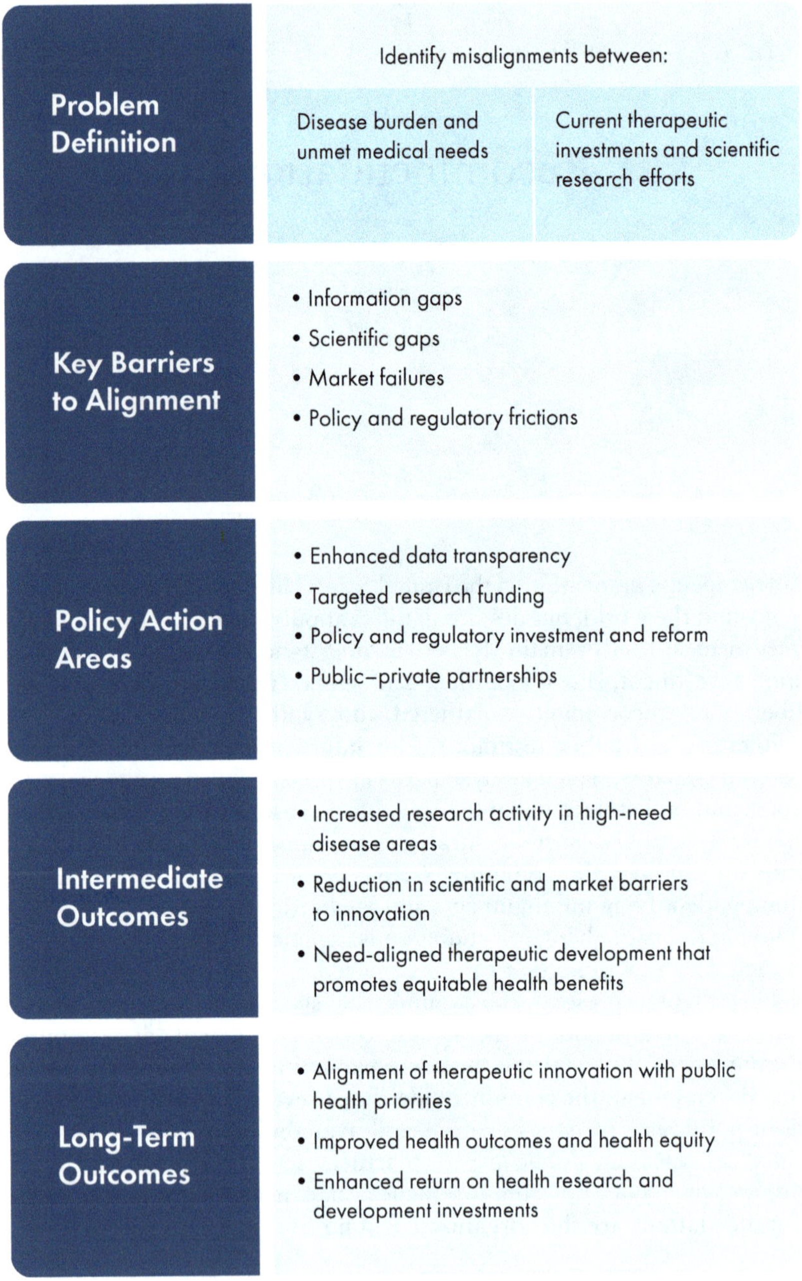

Problem Definition

Identify misalignments between:

| Disease burden and unmet medical needs | Current therapeutic investments and scientific research efforts |

Key Barriers to Alignment

- Information gaps
- Scientific gaps
- Market failures
- Policy and regulatory frictions

Policy Action Areas

- Enhanced data transparency
- Targeted research funding
- Policy and regulatory investment and reform
- Public–private partnerships

Intermediate Outcomes

- Increased research activity in high-need disease areas
- Reduction in scientific and market barriers to innovation
- Need-aligned therapeutic development that promotes equitable health benefits

Long-Term Outcomes

- Alignment of therapeutic innovation with public health priorities
- Improved health outcomes and health equity
- Enhanced return on health research and development investments

FIGURE 6-1 Conceptual framework work aligning investment with therapeutic need.

2. Support and strengthen public investment in innovative therapeutics that address unmet need.
3. Strengthen public–private partnerships to encourage the sharing of information and technology transfer to facilitate addressing unmet need.
4. Strengthen a regulatory environment that supports innovation to address unmet need.
5. Strengthen a fiscal and policy environment to align reimbursement policy with evidence-based therapeutic value and the extent to which products address unmet need.

In the rest of this chapter, each goal is discussed in turn, with recommendations made to a variety of key policy makers and decision makers in the therapeutic development landscape. The committee emphasizes specific, high-level actions needed to drive change by aligning incentives across multiple sectors that all play a role in drug development. Addressing each goal alone can mitigate a mismatch between investment in therapeutic development with unmet need, but when implemented in concert, these recommended actions will reinforce one another to drive meaningful change and bring to market effective therapies that address critical unmet needs.

GOAL 1: DESIGN A STATE-OF-THE-ART PUBLICLY ACCESSIBLE SYSTEM TO ASSESS AND TRACK UNMET NEED ASSOCIATED WITH U.S. DISEASE BURDEN, WITH A CRITICAL FOCUS ON IDENTIFYING AREAS OF MISMATCH AND REDUCING HEALTH DISPARITIES

Biomedical research is critical for improving the health of individuals worldwide. For millions of patients and their families, biomedical research provides hope for those dealing with life threatening and chronic diseases. Although research and innovation is not a zero-sum game, the resources available are unable to address all current health and research needs in a timely manner. Therefore, it is critical that there is a system in place that makes it possible to set research priorities and make difficult decisions about what funding is available to address health needs. As discussed in Chapter 3, these decisions are difficult and involve value judgments for prioritizing. While these value judgments are political decisions that may shift with changes in administrations or leadership in organizations, there is currently a lack of data with which leaders can make evidence-based policy judgments. Therefore, without the data necessary to assess how investments in therapeutic development align with disease burden and unmet need, research prioritization cannot be done accurately or effectively.

While various data sources provide insight into disease burden through common metrics like incidence, prevalence, and disability-adjusted life-years (DALYs), this information is not systematically compiled, nor is it regularly updated, analyzed, and used for the purpose of prioritizing needs. Having a way to systematically collect these data would further improve efficiency and effectiveness in decision making, as it reduces the number of demands on federal agencies and institutes to share how research priorities are set. Moreover, disease burden is multidimensional (see Chapter 2), suggesting the need for a more comprehensive and coordinated characterization of burden and need. This information gap makes it difficult to optimize investment in research. Without these data, public research funds are being allocated each year with insufficient information about the extent to which the investment is aligned with health needs.

A publicly accessible, centralized system to aggregate relevant data and track unmet medical need associated with disease burden would enable more strategic investment of resources and would help policy makers and public and private funding groups better align innovation and investment with health needs. This system could be used to identify disease areas to prioritize investment. These data could highlight areas of mismatch between investment and disease burden—including both conditions that need greater attention and those where there is overinvestment compared with relative burden. Existing models that could inform the development of such a system are the Institute for Health Metrics and Evaluation (IHME) Global Burden of Disease (GBD) Compare tool and Impact Global Health G-Finder project, both of which host the types of data that would need to be incorporated into the centralized system (IHME, 2025; Impact Global Health, 2024).

Developing standardized categories of disease and therapeutic areas for use in the system would help to enable comparisons between disease burden and investments in order to identify areas of mismatch. Similarly, methods that promote data transparency and accessibility, such as open methodologies, will facilitate a more comprehensive analysis of disease burden and unmet need. Because there will be several areas of mismatch that differ along a variety of relevant factors, such as the age of the affected population, disease acuity versus chronicity, and quality-of-life impact, the committee recognizes that it would be impossible to generate a single, universal list of priorities, as discussed in depth in Chapter 3. Instead, providing accessible data on burden, need, and current measures of public and private investment would enable public and private funders to make informed decisions based on their priorities and values. For example, some may prioritize rare, low-prevalence diseases with high individual burden, while others prioritize diseases with high population burden or high health disparities.

Developing this system is challenging. For instance, both burden and unmet need are difficult to define (see the committee's selected definitions in Chapter 2) and must be carefully considered in designing this system. Similarly, current investments are difficult to track, especially in the private sector. In addition, while some data are readily available and could be aggregated for this purpose, the committee recognizes that not all the data described in the recommendation are currently or easily accessible. To advance public health and reduce health disparities, these data should be collected, and it is important to invest in doing so.

Finally, it is important that these data be made public to the extent possible. There has been recent reporting about critical datasets and web pages being pulled from federal health websites, some of which is back online but with key data missing; such missing information damages scientists' ability to advance their research (Stone and Huang, 2025). Furthermore, given that these data are collected using public resources and do not contain proprietary information, it is critical that they remain accessible to the public. Therefore, recognizing that some information on private-sector investments may need to be aggregated to avoid sharing proprietary information, it is critical that the information collected on evaluating disease burden, unmet need, and the areas of investment be publicly available for all to use.

Finding 3-2: There are some existing data on disease burden, unmet need, and investment; however, these data are not regularly compiled and synthesized for assessing mismatch across factors. In addition, existing data are sometimes insufficient and have significant gaps. As a result, this committee lacked the data needed to produce a report that evaluates all aspects of disease burden, unmet need, and investment to fully assess the mismatch.

Finding 6-1: Disease burden and unmet need are multidimensional and challenging to measure, which suggests the need for multiple measures to effectively assess alignment or mismatch among these factors. A data repository that compiles multiple metrics of disease burden and unmet need would enable different organizations to access relevant data and create lists that reflect their priorities and values. For example, prioritizing reducing disparities across populations would require information on individual burden or data aggregated by relevant sociodemographic groups, not only population burden.

Finding 3-1: Characterizing past, current, and future priorities for investments in therapeutic innovation is multidimensional and complicated, especially given the longitudinal nature of research and development. Many of the data needed for this purpose are not publicly available. Some high-level data on industry investment are available, but the granularity of this information is limited.

Conclusion 3-1: More comprehensive, specific, timely, and accurate data on disease burden, unmet need, and innovation, as well as improved data aggregation, are essential for private and public funders to systematically use measures of disease burden and unmet need when making decisions about funding priorities.

Conclusion 3-2: Collecting and aggregating these data requires ongoing stewardship to most effectively address unmet clinical need and reduce health disparities.

Conclusion 3-3: The U.S. government has a responsibility to ensure that timely data on public investment and population health data be made publicly available to support research and strategic investment in areas of unmet need.

Recommendation 1: Congress should establish and fund an interagency consortium charged with tracking and assessing unmet therapeutic need associated with U.S. disease burden and current investments in innovation, with a critical focus on identifying areas of mismatch and reducing health disparities. The consortium should be led by a relevant unit of the Department of Health and Human Services (HHS) as determined by the Secretary of HHS.

This consortium should be charged with the following:

a. Generate a publicly accessible data repository on disease burden, therapeutic investment, and unmet needs that is updated on a triennial basis and used to generate derivative reports.

b. Produce a triennial report to Congress on the status of U.S. disease burden, extent of unmet need, and areas in which additional data are needed to reliably assess burden and unmet need. This report should collate, at minimum, for each disease area the current and projected incidence, prevalence, mortality, and disability-adjusted life-years.

c. Produce a companion assessment of the most reliable current estimates of investments from the public and private sectors for each therapeutic area, including public-sector funding by type and amount; private-sector investments; stage of the development pipeline for emerging treatments (e.g., drug discovery, preclinical research, clinical trials, regulatory review and approval, postapproval surveillance); the number, phase, and status of clinical trials; and sources of funding.

d. Identify areas in which additional research is needed to provide any missing information for each item above and recommending ways, such as statutory requirements or surveys, by which the data could be gathered for subsequent reports.

In addition to the data listed above, the triennial report to Congress would ideally contain additional information for each therapeutic area. For example, the report should include multiple additional measures of population burden and unmet need, such as years of life lost, equal value of life-years gained, and patient-reported outcomes. It should also include an assessment of individual burden, incorporating both patient and care-giver perspectives. The report should also list populations affected by age and at-risk subgroups that are disproportionately burdened, and current level of residual unmet need based on available treatments. The committee suggests categorizing unmet need by (a) no treatment exists, (b) treatment exists but is limited in its ability to address disease burden, overall or for specific at-risk subgroups of the population; (c) effective treatment exists, but access is limited: and (d) effective treatment exists and is accessible for all in need (i.e., no unmet need).

To implement this recommendation most effectively, it is critical that this consortium involve cross-agency and cross-disciplinary collaborators. Ideally, the following federal agencies and offices should be represented:[1] the Food and Drug Administration (FDA), National Institutes of Health (NIH), Centers for Disease Control and Prevention (CDC), the Office of the Assistant Secretary for Planning and Evaluation (ASPE), Office of the Assistant Secretary for Health, Assistant Secretary for Technology Policy, Advanced Research Projects Agency for Health (ARPA-H), Agency for Healthcare Research and Quality, Health Resources Services Administration, Indian Health Services, Centers for Medicare and Medicaid Services (CMS), the Department of Veterans Affairs, and the Department of Defense. ASPE, or another relevant office, may be a good fit to lead the organization of the consortium. In addition, the consortium should engage other key partners, including the Patient-Centered Outcomes Research Institute (PCORI) as well as industry organizations such as Pharmaceutical Research and Manufacturers of America (PhRMA) and Biotechnology Innovation Organization (BIO), and establish mechanisms to incorporate patient input, such as public comment periods or public meetings.

It is important for this consortium not only to collate these data but also to analyze and synthesize data, including identifying gaps and approaches for addressing these gaps. As an example, information about private-sector investment is not necessarily readily available. Although FDA requires that sponsors register trials in ClinicalTrials.gov, which may provide some insights into industrial areas of investment, sponsors are not required to

---

[1] At the time of publishing, the HHS agencies and offices listed here are still in operation. However, the committee recognizes that some of these agencies and offices may be part of an ongoing reorganization within HHS. Therefore, any similar office or agency that replaces the duties of the agencies or offices outlined here should be included in the cross-agency effort.

report phase I trials or small feasibility studies. Furthermore, there are often data missing, and researchers and investigators alike report difficulties using ClinicalTrials.gov (Chaturvedi et al., 2019; CTTI, 2024). ClinicalTrials.gov also does not provide insights into investment dollars that are spent on certain therapeutic areas.

Given the challenge of collecting information on private industry investments, the committee recognizes that companies may need to be incentivized to share or disclose some of these data that are not now publicly available. One way of collecting this information could be through a survey of pharmaceutical and biotech companies, which, while imperfect, could gather a useful sampling of data to gain insight into private investment in therapeutic development. An approach for incentivizing the collection of these data would be to delay public access for a period of time (e.g., 6 months) and allow early access to those companies that have contributed data. These data would provide a valuable, precompetitive resource that companies could use to make decisions and justifications for their intended actions. Some organizations, including the American Association for the Advancement of Science, IQVIA, and LEK Consulting, already report on private investment based on survey data. Similarly, data collected by the Association of University Technology Managers (AUTM) could be used to track investment from university venture funds. These data could be incorporated in the tracking system and reported in an aggregated and anonymized format and would still prove useful for understanding the landscape of private investment.

Although the consortium would ideally be housed within the federal government, the consortium might also exist with a trusted entity outside of the federal government. For example, the Foundation for the NIH (FNIH), an independent nonprofit organization, was recently contracted to be a trusted data broker between the private and public sector, on behalf of NIH, to develop a data access platform to implement the NIH's Data Counts program (TAGGS, 2024). If successful, this could potentially be a model to implement for this consortium.

Another challenge, which is nuanced, is assessing disease burden. As noted above, population burden is multifaceted. Ideally, a system for assessing disease burden should include multiple metrics to enable insight into different aspects of burden; however, this information is often incomplete or unavailable. Moreover, population burden alone does not provide a complete picture of disease burden; individual patient and caregiver burden offers an important counterpart. In some cases, such as in rare diseases, a condition may have low prevalence but high individual burden and high unmet need. Efforts to assess and measure individual (and caregiver) burden should incorporate patient perspectives without overburdening patients and communities.

There are also challenges in considering how new technologies could potentially shift how we think about disease burden. Previously, disease burden was thought about as burden that is avertable and burden that is inevitable. However, new technologies, like cell and gene therapies and other platform technologies, have made some inevitable burdens into avertable disease burdens. Therefore, although these considerations are not part of disease burden, it is important that some funding be considered for larger platform technologies that can shift innovation in substantial ways.

GOAL 2: SUPPORT AND STRENGTHEN INVESTMENTS IN INNOVATIVE THERAPEUTICS THAT ADDRESS UNMET NEED

The establishment of a comprehensive system to track and assess disease burden and unmet need, as recommended in Goal 1, should directly inform public and private investment in medical research and development. Congress plays a key role in defining the parameters of public investment in medical research by setting appropriations among the institutes and centers of NIH. Information about burden and unmet need should be incorporated at key points of decision making and should be an important resource for determining congressional appropriations and funding decisions at NIH and at other federal agencies. Private funders, including philanthropic organizations, should also consider these factors when making decisions about their funding priorities. While some private funders, such as foundations, may have a particular focus or goals, these factors can still be useful in guiding investment decisions within their areas that overlap with their mission.

However, considering burden and unmet need should not be limited to high-level priority setting. It should be integrated throughout the research funding process, from program development to grant review criteria, ensuring that unmet need is considered alongside scientific merit in such grant mechanisms. For example, ARPA-H could consider developing new programs specifically focused on the areas of highest mismatch between unmet need and investment. FDA could work with other agencies to advance development and validation of biomarkers. NIH could also do more to integrate these principles in its Small Business Innovation Research and Small Business Technology Transfer (SBIR/STTR) programs by prioritizing higher-risk, potentially revolutionary ventures that could address unmet needs and prioritize therapeutic development sources that are not covered by other investment sources. Furthermore, recognizing that NIH staff, such as the Council of Councils, is closer to understanding how unmet needs could be met with research funding, there should be some funding that they have discretion to allocate, with consideration for disease burden and unmet need. This could include Congress appropriating more funding with flexibility to be directed toward areas of highest unmet need and underinvestment, such as through the NIH Common Fund. This holistic approach would help align incentives to encourage investigators to consider unmet need early in the research process.

When funding agencies elevate the goal of addressing unmet need as a priority, researchers are more likely to develop studies to target these areas, leading to better alignment of public investment in medical research with public health needs.

> Recommendation 2: Funders of biomedical research should consider disease burden and unmet need when setting research priorities and directing funding. Specific actions to ensure both population health needs and scientific merit are considered in grant funding mechanisms include:
>
> a. Congress should consider disease burden and unmet needs when setting appropriations to agencies that fund biomedical research, including in allocating funding among National Institutes of Health institutes and centers.
> b. Public and private funders should develop targeted research funding opportunities specific to diseases with the highest mismatch of burden and unmet need, including funding opportunities for innovative methods to enable the development of therapeutic products and new biomarkers for diagnostic test development in these areas.
> c. Public and private funders should allocate funds for the development and validation of new biomarkers and surrogate endpoints for diseases with high unmet medical need.
> d. Public and private funders should provide funding for studies of disease epidemiology or basic science for areas where there is a critical need for understanding the mechanisms of disease.
> e. Public and private funders should include explicit criteria that include, but are not limited to, unmet need and disease burden for evaluating proposals in the grant review process and funding decisions.

The committee recognizes that NIH recently simplified peer-review criteria, and the "Importance of the Research" factor includes *significance* and *innovation* (NIH, 2024). However, incorporating unmet need and disease burden into reviewers' scoring can be achieved without major revision or complication. For example, NIH guidance on defining *significance* could be revised to make clear it includes social significance in addition to scientific significance. Alternatively, a separate high-level heading could be added to "Importance of the Research" to focus on social significance, such as unmet need and disease burden.

GOAL 3: STRENGTHEN PUBLIC–PRIVATE PARTNERSHIPS TO ENCOURAGE THE SHARING OF INFORMATION AND TECHNOLOGY TRANSFER TO FACILITATE ADDRESSING UNMET NEED

Goal 2 focused on the importance of public-sector actions to address disease burden and unmet need in funding decisions, but it is also important that the private sector takes these factors into account when developing a therapeutic portfolio. Generally, industry is constantly assessing unmet need to develop products that are most likely to generate returns on capital. However, as reviewed in Chapter 4, there are therapeutic areas where there is not a strong business case for developing an asset, or where an asset has been shelved for reasons unrelated to therapeutic potential. One way to develop these shelved assets that may address an unmet need is to develop and expand public–private partnerships (PPPs).

As discussed in Chapter 5, the committee defines PPPs as any type of cost or risk sharing between the public sector (both government and academia) and the private sector (private and public sources of capital, along with small and large industry). This includes bilateral government funding and legal mechanisms, such as cooperative research and development agreements (CRADAs), as well as larger multistakeholder projects between government, industry, academia, and nonprofits, such as those conducted by the congressionally authorized nonprofit organizations paired with the government scientific agencies.

Many strong global examples of PPPs are working to incentivize investment in areas of high disease burden and unmet need, including the Innovative Health Initiative in the European Union and the Global Health Innovative Technology Fund. The United States also has a number of PPP programs, described in detail in Chapter 5, such as Accelerating Medicines Partnerships (AMP), the Network for Excellence in Neuroscience Clinical Trials (NeuroNEXT), the National Cancer Institute Experimental Therapeutics (NExT) program, and Bridging Interventional Development Gaps (BrIDGs), that provide nondilutive funding for preclinical and clinical development. These programs are typically not focused on developing therapeutics that will benefit only one company or organization with its return on investment. However, they can be particularly useful for innovation in areas where cost and risk sharing are necessary, such as for novel drug target discovery, biomarker test development, or preclinical development models.

PPPs can be better used to address the misalignment for therapeutic areas where cost-sharing mechanisms can help address important unmet needs that are currently not being met owing to market disincentives. The committee is particularly interested in the potential for PPPs to fill three areas of unmet needs: (1) expanding the development of better diagnostics, which, as discussed in Chapter 4, is an area that is difficult to get funded by private-sector investment because of payment structures for diagnostic tests; (2) limiting situations where therapies that are effective and meeting an unmet need are taken off the market or where assets demonstrating early signs of efficacy are shelved before making it to market; and (3) providing an avenue for the development of drugs for diseases where there exists no economic incentive for the private sector to develop therapeutics.

As discussed in Chapter 4, diagnostics can efficiently and precisely identify the patients most likely to benefit from therapy, leading to more approvals of drugs that are safer and more effective. However, the payment structure for diagnostics is complicated and there are limited incentives for companies to develop diagnostics, unless they are linked directly to a therapeutic, such as with companion diagnostics. Furthermore, FDA approval for diagnostic tests require both analytical and clinical validation, and CMS may consider evidence of improved outcomes, or clinical utility, when the test is used, in determining coverage and reimbursement of the diagnostic. Such outcome studies can be lengthy and thus costly. Therefore, despite the potential for diagnostics to address unmet needs and to facilitate accurate diagnosis for drug development for unmet health needs, incentives to innovate in this space are lacking. As a result, the committee believes that PPPs could be one way to develop better diagnostics, such as for some elements of generating evidence supportive of patient access. As noted in Chapter 5, PPPs are often most effective when focusing on the precompetitive space, such as developing better biomarkers. Therefore, this could be a useful area for PPPs to focus and drive innovation for unmet needs.

PPPs could also be particularly useful in keeping effective therapeutics meeting an unmet need on the market when there is a threat of them being pulled. For example, Novo Nordisk recently discontinued a long-acting insulin, Levemir, in part because of market forces (Alltucker, 2024). In a congressional hearing focused on the decision to pull Levemir from the market, the CEO of Novo Nordisk said the company would be willing to share the drug's formulation with other manufacturers, including the U.S. government. As discussed in Chapter 5, there are many private businesses that work to obtain abandoned assets from other companies to develop. The committee is not proposing that PPPs could replace these industries, but they would fill in gaps where either the financing model is not favorable because of risk or the market dynamics do not make the asset desirable. By using nonprofit organizations for the federal agencies, such as the Foundation for the NIH and the Reagan-Udall Foundation, federal health agencies could work to continue manufacturing therapeutics in such situations so patients gain access to effective therapeutics for the public good, even when there is not a profitable market for industry.

Finally, PPPs could be useful for developing drugs in therapeutic areas where little to no economic incentives exist for the private sector. Chapter 4 outlines several reasons why market forces prevent innovation in areas of unmet need, including small patient sizes and limited applicability of therapeutics. PPPs could be used to provide creative sources of financing to develop therapeutics in these areas and thus advance innovation where potential profits are limited.

Finding 5-11: PPPs can effectively enable the private sector to share both costs and risks.

Finding 5-3: Addressing unmet clinical need sometimes requires novel diagnostic tests to characterize diseases and disease states. For example, novel drugs often depend on accurate diagnostics to identify who should receive the treatment.

Finding 4-2: Despite early signs of efficacy or even FDA approval of a drug, some therapeutics are shelved or pulled from the market because there is not a large enough economic incentive or return on investment for a company to fully develop the drug or continue manufacturing it once approved.

Finding 5-12: Every scientific health research agency has a congressionally mandated nonprofit organization that could be useful in building PPPs.

Conclusion 5-1: Diagnostics to characterize and detect disease states are critical for developing innovative therapies, targeting therapeutics to those who will benefit, and ensuring that patients have access to therapeutics early enough in their disease progression for therapeutics to be effective, and they are an important component of addressing unmet clinical need. Further incentives for development of innovative and accurate diagnostic tests that are necessary for drugs that address unmet medical needs could help resolve the mismatch among therapeutic investment, disease burden, and unmet need.

Conclusion 5-9: Strengthening and expanding public–private partnerships, such as the Network for Excellence in Neuroscience Clinical Trials, the National Cancer Institute Experimental Therapeutics program, and Bridging Interventional Development Gaps, could help address innovation challenges for therapeutic areas with unmet needs.

Recommendation 3: U.S. federal scientific agencies with congressionally authorized nonprofit organizations, such as the Foundation for the National Institutes of Health, Centers for Disease Control and Prevention Foundation, Reagan-Udall Foundation, and Henry M. Jackson Foundation for the Advancement of Military Medicine, should increase use of their nonprofits in order to focus on building public–private partnerships in areas of mismatch between unmet need (encompassing both therapeutics and diagnostics) and innovation.

Despite the many successes of PPPs, as discussed in Chapter 5, federal agencies do not always have insight into what shelved assets exist in pharmaceutical companies and therefore are unable to approach companies about developing these assets. Therefore, having an independent organization house a searchable repository of assets to which companies voluntarily submit information could help overcome this barrier. The committee recognizes that some companies may not be willing to share this information. However, it could be used by other industries looking to purchase a shelved asset, which may bring profits to industries looking to offload assets.

There may also be concerns about liability in selling an asset to a PPP or to another company. While outside the scope of this committee, it may be worth further attention to mitigate potential liability either through indemnification or other statutory measures. This repository might not be publicly available in order to safeguard proprietary information, but it would be viewable by federal agencies, other foundations, companies, and nonprofits that apply for access. Although it likely would not contain a complete list of shelved assets, it would be a start for advancing PPPs in areas of unmet need and where the market does not support further innovation.

The New Therapeutic Uses program from the National Center for Advancing Translational Sciences (NCATS) aims to accomplish some of this by focusing on drug repurposing. However, the New Therapeutic Uses program focuses on repurposing already approved drugs for other conditions, rather than assets under development. Furthermore, it does not appear that awards have been granted through this program since 2021, indicating the need for additional resources toward this goal.

Although created for different purposes, the National Cancer Institute (NCI) Formulary is a PPP between NCI and pharmaceutical and biotechnology companies where the companies volunteer assets that have shown promise in preclinical testing to be tested by NCI-funded investigators. Although the purpose of this specific PPP is to expedite investigator access to therapeutics in clinical trials and not necessarily to host a list of searchable assets, the success of the NCI Formulary could lay the groundwork for a more generalized searchable repository.

Recommendation 4: The National Institutes of Health should work with a neutral third-party entity to set up a searchable repository of assets no longer under development by commercial sponsors to be shared with foundations and other entities to take forward for testing. The information in the repository could be voluntarily provided by companies potentially looking to enter public–private partnerships to develop an asset.

Another barrier to successful PPPs, as discussed in Chapter 5, is the absence of a "warm" clinical trial infrastructure that is ready to go. Often, clinical trial networks are set up, only to be disbanded when a specific project ends because funding does not exist to sustain the staffing or infrastructure. Currently, industry does not typically use these public networks (outside of NCI) because many of the contractual and intellectual property elements are not viewed as favorable by the private sector. For example, one area of friction between industry and academia in the precompetitive space arises over intellectual property (Perkmann et al., 2011). This can be seen in one form in partnerships where academics are using company assets. Academic researchers are accustomed to freely publishing results, and academic research institutions have their own appetite for entrepreneurship. However, industry is often concerned with intellectual property (IP) protections and regulatory filings and are not eager to share data or results on the timelines desired by academics. This is especially true for highly novel assets being tested clinically.

The clinical trial infrastructure set up by NIH institutes involves academic researchers and institutions in addition to government. This can cause even more complex disagreements over IP between government, company, and academic institution policies being in conflict and creating a barrier to setting up effective PPPs due to the necessary complex negotiations. Even the simplest bilateral partnerships between NIH and industry can encounter difficulties. Currently, each NIH institute has its own rules for developing CRADAs for these PPPs. Some institutes, such as NCI, are more sympathetic to IP concerns, while other institutes require more data sharing. This lack of standardized contractual frameworks across NIH often results in confusion about entering into CRADAs and difficulties in negotiating the CRADAs across institutes. Therefore, having an established set of contractual and IP frameworks across NIH that protects patients' interest in access to the resulting products could potentially expedite PPPs. The committee recognizes that there may be circumstances where different frameworks are desired, such as during a public health emergency, so the committee recommends a set of frameworks that accounts for these scenarios.

Recommendation 5: The director of the National Institutes of Health (NIH) should establish a set of contractual and intellectual property frameworks for industry allowing greater incentivization and smoother use of the NIH clinical trials infrastructure that balances the interests of NIH, NIH-funded investigators and their institutions, patients, and industry partners.

GOAL 4: STRENGTHEN A REGULATORY ENVIRONMENT THAT SUPPORTS INNOVATION TO ADDRESS UNMET NEED

Chapter 4 of this report details the challenges that lead to a misalignment of innovations with disease burden and unmet need. One of the challenges causing a misalignment is a lack of understanding of the underlying pathophysiology of many diseases. Without an understanding of how diseases work and how therapeutics could potentially target those diseases, innovation is unlikely to advance. As the committee heard throughout its public sessions, life science investors and industry scientists depend on advances in basic and preclinical biomedical research to attract their attention and funding. And, as described in Chapter 5, too often the problem facing patients is not that FDA is standing in the way of good drugs, but that there are not enough good drugs moving their way through the research and development process. Therefore, advancing basic and preclinical research in disease areas with a high disease burden and high unmet needs would improve innovation and reduce therapeutic gaps.

Finding 4-1: Investment in basic and preclinical biomedical research is essential to driving innovation in disease areas with significant disease burden that have unmet needs.

In the committee's analysis of reasons for misalignment between investment in therapeutic development and unmet need, it did not find that the misalignment was caused by action or inaction from FDA. Although FDA sometimes is cited as a barrier to innovation, the committee did not find evidence to support this claim.

Finding 5-2: Many of the current drivers contributing to the misalignment of innovation and investment with disease burden and unmet need are not within FDA's immediate control.

Furthermore, as outlined in Chapter 5, FDA has several ongoing programs to drive and support innovation in much-needed areas. These programs generally fall into three categories: (1) efforts to encourage investment to address unmet need; (2) efforts to address broad scientific challenges, improve coordination, and encourage data generation to address unmet need; and (3) efforts to facilitate and expedite development, review, and approval to address unmet need.

Chapter 5 reviews a number of FDA programs designed to encourage investment in certain disease areas. Although there are differing opinions on the efficacy of some of these programs, particularly for priority review vouchers, there was not sufficient evidence to support expanding these programs to address unmet needs.

Finding 5-4: Whether or not the Orphan Drug Act (ODA) is narrowed or otherwise adjusted, there is no convincing evidence to suggest that the recent growth in rare disease innovation is a result of ODA incentives.

Finding 5-5: Without taking a position on whether priority review voucher programs should be renewed, the committee finds no convincing evidence to suggest that they should be expanded as a tool to better match investment and unmet need.

Conclusion 5-2: The committee did not find sufficient evidence to recommend expansion of priority review vouchers, orphan drug exclusivity, or patent term extensions in their current form to support drug development to better meet unmet needs.

As for the second category of FDA programs that address broad scientific challenges, improve coordination, and encourage data generation to address unmet needs, many of these programs are pilot programs or have only been in place for a short time. Therefore, there is not yet sufficient evidence to recommend expansion of these programs. However, the committee strongly supports the ideas behind these programs, many of which are intended to improve science and expedite innovation without lowering safety or efficacy standards.

Finding 5-6: Because FDA programs to address broad scientific challenges, with the exception of pediatric study requirements, have only been in place for a few years, it will be important to carefully evaluate their effect and resource burdens, both individually and collectively, and to devote additional resources to successful programs.

Finding 5-9: Through a wide range of programs, FDA has demonstrated creativity and commitment to supporting the science necessary for successful drug development and to providing regulatory support for sponsors seeking to address unmet need, especially in the context of rare disease.

Conclusion 5-3: Additional resources are needed for FDA programs that successfully support endpoint development and validation, innovative trial design, and the resolution of other broad scientific challenges that impede drug development for unmet needs, as well as programs designed to support communication between sponsors and FDA to quickly resolve challenges arising in specific development programs.

The last category of FDA programs is intended to facilitate and expedite the development and review of new therapeutics to address unmet needs, including through heightened regulatory support, shortened review periods, and alternative approaches to demonstrating effectiveness, thereby encouraging industry investment in these areas.

Finding 5-10: FDA has several programs designed to drive innovation in therapeutic areas of unmet need, including the breakthrough therapy and fast track designations, priority review, and accelerated approval, as well as less formal approaches to regulatory flexibility.

The most controversial of these programs has been the accelerated approval pathway, which accepts uncertainty regarding a drug's clinical benefit in exchange for early approval, with the expectation that benefit will be established through postapproval confirmatory studies. In response to a number of concerns about confirmatory study delay, one of the goals of the 2022 Food and Drug Omnibus Reform Act (FDORA) was to improve the timely completion of confirmatory studies following accelerated approval. FDORA affirms FDA's discretionary authority to require confirmatory studies be underway before approval is granted (FDA, 2025), which has been demonstrated to improve timely completion and conversion to regular approval (Fashoyin-Aje et al., 2022), though timely studies may not be feasible in extreme cases, such as ultrarare diseases. FDORA also created a requirement that sponsors submit more frequent progress reports on confirmatory studies (now every 6 months instead of annually) and requires that these reports be published on the agency's website. Because these programs were recently enacted, it is premature to evaluate success, although they are strong steps toward promoting timeliness, especially given known challenges that make recruitment and retention difficult for confirmatory studies once patients can access approved drugs on the market.

In addition to timely completion of confirmatory studies following accelerated approval, it is also important to ensure that accelerated approval is granted only when drugs truly are reasonably likely to demonstrate clinical benefit (i.e., based on appropriate surrogate endpoints), that confirmatory studies are rigorously designed in addition to being completed on time, and that drugs whose studies fail to clearly confirm clinical benefit are quickly withdrawn. Yet, evidence indicates concern in each of these domains: FDA has sometimes accepted controversial surrogate endpoints to support accelerated approval (Largent et al., 2022; McIntyre, 2024); confirmatory studies often lack important features of rigorous design, such as being conducted without randomization or a control group or continuing to rely on surrogate endpoints (Gyawali et al., 2019; Naci et al., 2017; Sachs et al., 2022); and drugs are sometimes converted to regular approval even when they fail to confirm benefit (Gyawali et al., 2021).

Although FDORA included provisions to require that key confirmatory study design parameters be established no later than the point of accelerated approval and to potentially expedite withdrawal proceedings when initiated by FDA, neither the law nor subsequent FDA guidance has sufficiently clarified the level of appropriate flexibility in accepting new surrogate endpoints to support accelerated approval, addressed poor rigor in confirmatory study design, or addressed FDA's response when confirmatory studies fail to clearly demonstrate a drug's clinical benefit. Therefore, these concerns remain unresolved, jeopardizing the promise and success of the accelerated approval program. In addition, although FDA has a Biomarker Qualification Program intended to support the identification and development of new biomarkers and to qualify biomarkers for specific contexts of use (FDA, 2021), sponsors have little incentive to undertake the necessary studies as they are complex and expensive, and qualification is not a required condition of using biomarkers to support approval.

Conclusion 5-4: Given important concerns about the accelerated approval pathway, recent adjustments need to be carefully monitored and further adjustments may be needed to promote rigor and confidence that accelerated approval drugs will, as quickly as is possible, confirm meaningful clinical benefit for patients or be withdrawn.

Conclusion 5-5: Current legislation and polices for FDA are sufficient to foster the approval of innovative drugs for unmet needs.

Recommendation 6: To maintain the appropriateness of Food and Drug Administration (FDA) programs that expedite the development and review of therapies in areas of unmet need, including the accelerated approval program, FDA should generously use its authority to impose postmarket study requirements, ensure that required postmarket studies are appropriately designed to confirm clinical benefit, and strictly enforce postmarket study requirements. The following steps will support these goals:

a. **FDA should ensure that confirmatory studies are well designed to evaluate clinical benefit and should prespecify the study results that will be deemed acceptable for conversion to traditional approval.**

b. FDA should continue recent efforts to ensure that confirmatory studies are underway before approval is granted, making exceptions only in extreme cases.

c. If concerns about timely study completion arise during progress reports, then FDA and the sponsor should determine the steps needed to address barriers; any modification to study requirements should prioritize ensuring rigor.

d. For drugs whose studies fail to confirm clinical benefits following flexible approval, FDA should use its authority to rapidly withdraw approval.

e. FDA should lead an effort, in collaboration with the National Institutes of Health and the Centers for Medicare & Medicaid Services, to enable more efficient conversion of unvalidated endpoints to validated endpoints to advance therapeutic innovation.

Although it is not a specific program, FDA sometimes uses informal regulatory flexibility to expand patient access to therapeutics. This informal flexibility is applied to both accelerated approval products and to those receiving regular approval (see Chapter 5 for specific examples where FDA has used regulatory flexibility). Regulatory flexibility can be appropriate as long as there is strong reason to expect that clinical benefit will be confirmed later and those expectations are enforced by requiring that rigorous confirmatory studies be promptly completed.

As discussed in Chapter 5, FDA regulatory flexibility can include approval based on a single pivotal study, acceptance of single arm trials, acceptance of poor surrogate endpoints for accelerated approval, acceptance of surrogate endpoints outside accelerated approval, and approval despite trials missing prespecified endpoints, among other flexibilities. FDA acknowledges that for serious diseases, the agency may accept weaker trial designs and endpoints, fewer trials, or less statistical confidence, pointing to perceived patient "willingness to accept less certainty about effectiveness in return for earlier access to much needed medicines" (FDA, 2019).

Despite the substantial flexibility exercised both within the accelerated approval program and beyond it, some argue that FDA is still not flexible enough and that even greater regulatory flexibility is needed. The suggested solutions range from encouraging new regulatory flexibilities in certain cases, such as for rare diseases (Quandt, 2022; Woodcock et al., 2024), to calls for greater regulatory flexibility in general (Foundation for Government Accountability, 2022).

While greater regulatory flexibility can improve access to innovative therapeutics, there is an important balance between being appropriately flexible and weakening regulatory standards to such a great extent that patients and clinicians lose sufficient confidence that a drug will confer its purported benefit. For example, regulatory flexibility may be critical for disease areas, such as ultrarare diseases, where it is nearly impossible to meet standard expectations. However, when well-designed trials are completed but fail to demonstrate a benefit, approving the drug does not meet patient needs; unmet need is addressed by access to good, effective drugs, not simply by allowing more drugs on the market.

Weak approval standards risk harming patients in a variety of ways, including through a lack of adequate information necessary for patients and clinicians to make informed treatment decisions, possible exposure to side effects (and costs) not justified by benefits, and lost opportunity to participate in trials of alternative therapies or to pursue other treatment or palliation plans that may be more suitable. In addition, weak standards can inhibit innovation by impeding the conduct of clinical trials for new products by, for example slowing patient recruitment (as patients pursue the uncertain-but-approved product instead of trial participation) or by complicating study design through requiring comparison to an unproven standard of care. Most importantly, weak approval standards fail to incentivize true innovation for the benefit of patients, instead accepting unproven or weak clinical options.

In the case of regulatory flexibility, it is in the public's interest to maintain reasonably high standards for drug approval and when flexibility is offered, to ensure that benefit is confirmed after approval in a timely manner.

Finding 5-7: FDA currently exercises a great deal of regulatory flexibility both within and beyond existing programs and sometimes extends this flexibility too far by approving drugs that are unlikely to—or fail to—confirm benefit.

Finding 5-8: Given the remaining unmet need, FDA is under pressure to increase regulatory flexibility beyond current approaches.

Conclusion 5-6: When traditional approval standards cannot be satisfied for scientific reasons, regulatory flexibility can be appropriate as long as the initial approval is based on a reasonable likelihood of clinical benefit and clinical benefit is rigorously and rapidly confirmed following approval.

Conclusion 5-7: Although patients facing serious unmet needs may reasonably be willing to accept greater uncertainty and risk, weak approval standards harm patients seeking clear information to guide treatment decisions, may impede the development of strong treatment options, and fail to incentivize investment in true innovation.

Recommendation 7: To ensure that regulatory flexibility is exercised in a manner that promotes the approval of drugs that are both safe and effective, the Food and Drug Administration (FDA) should uphold strong regulatory approval standards. When FDA exercises flexibility, whether through accelerated approval or outside that pathway, the agency should require rigorous, timely confirmatory studies.

As discussed earlier in Chapter 5, FDA has a number of efforts underway to encourage investment to address unmet needs; to address broad scientific challenges, improve coordination, and encourage data generation to address unmet needs; and to facilitate and expedite development, review, and approval to address unmet needs. For FDA to maintain many of these pathways and initiatives, the agency requires appropriate funding and staffing. "FDA is a staff-intensive agency, with approximately 80 percent of its budget devoted to personnel costs" needed to appropriately recruit and retain individuals with the expertise needed to regulate food and drug products (NTEU, 2024). However, FDA has faced a number of concerning staff disruptions recently, including layoffs, retirements, forced resignations, and departures (Cranmer, 2024; Karlin-Smith, 2024; Lawrence, 2024; Lawrence and Feuerstein, 2025; Lawrence and Parker, 2025; Wilkerson, 2023), threatening the agency's ability to manage its intensive workload and advance innovative approaches (Hopkins, 2025).

Maintaining and expanding the FDA workforce is essential to allowing the agency to keep pace with technological and scientific breakthroughs (Deloitte, 2018). For example, holding frequent meetings between FDA staff and sponsors is critical to ensure that applications are as robust as possible. Even prior to recent layoffs, FDA needed additional support to advance innovation for areas of unmet need. With the recent layoffs and departures, and the associated uncertainty they have wrought for federal employees who already accept far less than they could earn in industry in order to support FDA's public health mission, it is unlikely that FDA will be able to maintain or expand its pilot programs helping spur research and expedite approval for needed therapeutics. Ultimately, without congressional action to adequately fund FDA and protect appropriate staffing levels, the agency will not be able to support the kind of workforce, in terms of expertise and experience, needed to advance therapeutic development for unmet needs.

Conclusion 5-8: Support for innovation in the pre- and postmarket settings requires a well-resourced regulatory environment, including attracting and retaining FDA staff with the necessary experience and expertise.

Recommendation 8: Congress should authorize a significant expansion of Food and Drug Administration (FDA) staffing and consistent resources to support the implementation of Recommendations 6 and 7, and especially to ensure that FDA has sufficient resources to monitor and enforce requirements for postmarketing surveillance and drug evaluation research.

GOAL 5: STRENGTHEN A FISCAL AND POLICY ENVIRONMENT TO ALIGN REIMBURSEMENT POLICY WITH EVIDENCE-BASED THERAPEUTIC VALUE AND THE EXTENT TO WHICH PRODUCTS ADDRESS UNMET NEED

The current U.S. drug pricing and reimbursement system creates strong incentives for innovation—particularly for novel therapies addressing unmet needs—but, at the same time, it may perpetuate inequitable access to effective treatments. Notably, the United States spends more on health care per capita than other high-income countries (Gunja et al., 2023; Peter G. Peterson Foundation, 2024; Wager et al., 2024), while not delivering commensurate levels of quality of outcomes.

Reimbursement policy through public (Medicare and Medicaid) and private plans (employer-sponsored and individual market health plans) determines whether a novel drug is covered and, if covered, the amount paid by beneficiaries. As reviewed in Chapter 4, disincentives for innovation can occur if novel drugs that address unmet need are not covered or are not readily accessible by patients through access restrictions, such as utilization management strategies or by cost-sharing (i.e., copay obligations) that is too high for patients to afford. In addition, providing high coverage and payment for therapies without demonstrated clinical benefit or substantive innovation undermines the potential of reimbursement policy to incentivize the development of high-value treatments over marginal improvements. One approach that may increase the clinical value of a product is through the development of diagnostics that can enable segmentation of a broader patient population for personalized medicine approaches. Aligning reimbursement policy with evidence-based value, of which unmet need must be a component, is key to this committee's aims of promoting innovation and addressing unmet need.

A revised approach to reimbursement policy could help address innovation incentives for therapeutic development by linking pricing to evidence-based value assessments that incorporate clinical effectiveness, patient perspectives, and assessments of unmet need. Several other countries offer useful models for this approach—prioritizing payment for new therapies that address unmet need and limiting reimbursement for products that offer marginal improvements or whose clinical benefit remains unproven. For example, the United Kingdom and Germany both have systems for evaluating the clinical effectiveness of a treatment to determine payment (Lemley et al., 2020). (See Chapter 5 for more information about reimbursement and payment policy.) Linking pricing to value is also important because prioritizing payment for high-value innovative therapies (while limiting overpaying for lower value treatments) could make more resources available for improving coverage for effective therapies. That is, coverage should also follow evidence.

Accordingly, there is an impetus to align reimbursement policy in a way that incentivizes companies to invest in innovative new therapies that provide value by addressing unmet need. Research indicates that pharmaceutical companies respond to financial incentives and direct innovation efforts toward areas with greater financial incentives (Hemel and Ouellette, 2023). Thus, this is a promising avenue to pursue.

Reforming reimbursement policy and incentivizing innovation to address unmet needs requires grappling with the definition and value assessment of *unmet need*. Value-based pricing can be implemented through different approaches, which need not be directly linked to unmet need. However, if the value of a new therapy is defined based on the benefits it provides relative to the current standard of care, then value will be aligned with the degree to which the therapy addresses unmet need. Societal value and addressing unmet need are thus mutually reinforcing concepts that are central to this committee's recommendations. Furthermore, a frequent criticism of aligning reimbursement policy with value is that it will lead to increased insurance premiums, resulting in fewer people buying insurance and getting access to therapeutics. Another criticism is that negotiating drug prices will make innovation more difficult or costly. However, in this report, the focus is on spending more efficiently on therapeutics, not spending more. This means redistributing spending to align better with the value of drugs that are available to patients, so that insurers are paying more for higher value drugs and less for lower value drugs. Therefore, net spending would be unchanged, but for the same amount of spending, more patients that need high value medicines would gain access.

Finding 5-13: An expectation of increased financial return for a certain class of pharmaceutical product has been shown to increase R&D effort on those products.

Finding 5-14: Many countries negotiate drug prices and set reimbursement terms based on the product's cost-effectiveness, including considerations of unmet need.

Finding 5-15: CMS has statutory authority to use comparative effectiveness and unmet medical needs for a limited number of older drugs under the Medicare price negotiation and New Technology Add-On Payment programs, but it otherwise lacks authority to control Medicare or Medicaid reimbursement amounts for most new drugs.

Conclusion 5-10: If public and private payer reimbursement policies were more aligned with evidence of product value and the extent to which a drug addresses unmet medical need, greater innovation would occur in therapeutic areas with high unmet need.

Conclusion 5-11: Congressional action is needed to more directly tie prices and public insurance reimbursement for novel drugs that address unmet need to evidence-supported measures of value or impact.

Recommendation 9: Congress should reform the statutory framework that regulates public reimbursement for novel drugs to better align reimbursement rates with evidence of clinical benefit as compared with existing therapeutic alternatives, if any. This could include:
a. Expand the Centers for Medicare & Medicaid Services' authority and capacity to negotiate prices beyond the scope of the Inflation Reduction Act to account for the value of the drug relative to alternatives or a standard of care, including the extent to which it addresses unmet need.
b. For drugs with negotiated prices, set reimbursement terms that maximize patient access through more favorable cost-sharing, robust formulary coverage, and more tailored application of utilization management tools (e.g., prior authorization, step-therapy, and quantity limits).

Recommendation 10: The Centers for Medicare & Medicaid Services should use its existing regulatory authority to reduce the mismatch between Medicare reimbursement for a drug and that drug's ability to address unmet medical needs, including through its implementation of the drug price negotiation program and the New Technology Add-on Payment program.

Although Recommendation 10 is targeted at CMS, the goal is for both public and private insurance systems to align payment with evidence of clinical benefit. However, because CMS is the largest single provider in the U.S. market, the prices it negotiates are likely to have ripple effects, affecting drug prices in the private market as well.

One-time, curative or regenerative medicine therapies face particular challenges in the current market and reimbursement system. Novel one-time, or limited duration curative, therapies have been developed in recent years but have often not easily reached patients, in part because of high up-front costs and the fragmented nature of U.S. health insurance coverage. Recent examples of such therapies have included treatments for beta thalassemia, immunologically driven diseases, and sickle cell anemia. With new developments in cell and gene therapies in recent years, the number of such therapies is increasing. It is important that these therapies continue to be developed—some are highly effective and innovative with the potential to revolutionize the future of targeted therapeutics for other conditions and provide long-term cost savings, but the market and access barriers are significant.

The benefit designs and utilization management employed by many insurance payers in the United States make it difficult for clinicians, individual patients and manufacturers, and innovators to navigate coverage and patient access for these very high-priced drugs. This has resulted in lower or no access to certain drugs, depending on insurance coverage and even geography (e.g., variation by states among Medicaid insured populations). Private market efforts to ameliorate these challenges, such as outcomes-based contracts, have not been broadly effective. Recent efforts by the Center for Medicare and Medicaid Innovation through its Cell and Gene Therapy Access Model targeting Medicaid coverage for sickle cell therapies reflect the growing recognition for the need of more consolidated efforts for determining reimbursement, market access, and data collection needs for these therapies.

Among commercially insured patients, access is also a challenge since smaller insurers and employers may be unable to afford the high costs of practically any of the curative therapies, and traditional sources of reinsurance and risk pooling may explicitly exclude coverage for these therapies (Phares et al., 2024). Even among larger employers, there may be resistance to covering high-cost therapies where benefits are perceived to accrue to future employers, insurance plans, or government payers.

Recent evidence also suggests that as product commercialization has, in some cases, underperformed investor expectations, new investments in cell and gene therapies and curative therapies are being challenged and drug developers have begun to retreat from this market. Given the exceptional benefits of these products for patients (and especially for those with very rare diseases), it is imperative to improve market access for these novel therapies that aim to address unmet needs. To improve affordability and access for patients and to sustain investments in these needed innovative treatments, novel solutions for payment, coverage, and market access for drug developers, payers, and patients are needed (Phares et al., 2024).

Conclusion 4-1: Innovative therapies are emerging for rare diseases and other complex conditions, offering a potential for cure. However, the fragmented payment system within the United States is a barrier to patient access, resulting in underinvestment in developing curative therapies. The current U.S. market and policy environment is unprepared to manage these one-time, very high-cost therapies. There is a need for a clearer reimbursement structure for innovators developing these high-cost curative treatments.

Recommendation 11: Congress should support the development of a negotiation and access model for one-time curative therapies to ensure access for patients and market access for innovators of novel therapies.

Congress should instruct an organization or agency, such as the Medicare Payment Advisory Commission or the Medicaid and CHIP Payment and Access Commission, to study and develop recommendations for legislation to create a new program addressing the unique deficiencies of the nation's current insurance system in enabling access to curative therapies. The details of designing this system are beyond the scope of this report, but several possibilities and considerations have been identified.

The program would likely be based on carving coverage of these therapies out of the myriad current insurance programs and into a new national risk pool that would serve as the source of coverage, access, and payment for these medicines. The program could be managed by either private entities or public, depending on the preferences of Congress. Sustainable fair prices would be negotiated by the administrating entity along with guidelines for appropriate access. The process for price benchmarking and negotiations will have to be defined and would likely benefit from the greatest possible transparency. The program design will need to contemplate the nature of the medicines eligible for inclusion, such as the size of the eligible population, the price of the treatment, the duration of treatment, and the curative success rate and sustainability, including evidentiary requirements. The program will likewise need to consider whether all such medicines are to be automatically enrolled or whether participation would be voluntary for both parties and so based on a successful negotiation of mutually satisfactory fair prices and fair access. Funding for the new program will also have to be developed. Some possibilities might include a new tax on insurance premiums making up for the carve out, a new Medicare tax, a new general income tax, or a new tax on generic medicines.

Medicare coverage through Social Security disability insurance could provide one potential pathway for access. For example, Medicare coverage could be expanded to include coverage for one-time curative therapies, similar to its coverage for individuals diagnosed with end-stage renal disease or amyotrophic lateral sclerosis. Coverage could be limited to a defined treatment episode for individuals insured by commercial or Medicaid payers. In addition, Medicare could use an approach to price negotiation similar to the one used under the Inflation Reduction Act, allowing for fair prices and fair access for drugs that otherwise may not reach patients under the status quo.

REFERENCES

Alltucker, K. 2024. Senate panel questions Novo Nordisk CEO over decision to discontinue this popular insulin. *USA Today*, September 25. https://www.usatoday.com/story/news/health/2024/09/25/novonordisk-ceo-levemir-insulin-discontinuation/75363969007/ (accessed January 15, 2025).

Chaturvedi, N., B. Mehrotra, S. Kumari, S. Gupta, H. S. Subramanya, and G. Saberwal. 2019. Some data quality issues at ClinicalTrials.Gov *Trials* 20(1):378.

Cranmer, J. 2024. Bob Temple, father of modern FDA, set to retire. *Biocentury*, December 19. https://www.biocentury.com/article/654528/bob-temple-father-of-modern-fda-set-to-retire (accessed January 15, 2025).

CTTI (Clinical Trials Transformation Initiative). 2024. *Improving timely, accurate, and complete registration and reporting of summary results information on ClinicalTrials.gov.* https://ctti-clinicaltrials.org/wp-content/uploads/2024/01/CTTI_SuggestedPractices_ClinicalTrials-gov_FINAL.pdf (accessed April 21, 2025).

Deloitte. 2018. *A bold future for life sciences regulation.* https://www.deloitte.com/cz-sk/en/Industries/life-sciences-health-care/analysis/life-sciences-predictions.html (accessed April 22, 2025).

Fashoyin-Aje, L. A., G. U. Mehta, J. A. Beaver, and R. Pazdur. 2022. The on- and off-ramps of oncology accelerated approval. *New England Journal of Medicine* 387(16):1439–1442.

FDA (Food and Drug Administration). 2019. *Demonstrating substantial evidence of effectiveness for human drug and biological products.* Draft guidance for industry. Docket no. FDA-2019-D-4964. https://www.fda.gov/regulatory-information/search-fda-guidance-documents/demonstrating-substantial-evidence-effectiveness-human-drug-and-biological-products (accessed April 22, 2025).

FDA. 2021. *About biomarkers and qualification.* https://www.fda.gov/drugs/biomarker-qualification-program/about-biomarkers-and-qualification#How_can_qualified_biomarkers_improve_the_drug_development_process (accessed May 16, 2025).

FDA. 2025. *Accelerated approval and considerations for determining whether a confirmatory trial is underway.* Silver Spring, MD: Food and Drug Administration. https://www.fda.gov/media/184831/download (accessed April 20, 2025).

Foundation for Government Accountability. 2022. *Frequently asked questions: Promising Pathway Act.* https://thefga.org/one-pagers/frequently-asked-questions-promising-pathway-act-h-r-3761-s-1644/ (accessed January 8, 2025).

Gunja, M. Z., E. D. Gumas, and R. D. Williams II. 2023. *U.S. health care from a global perspective, 2022: Accelerating spending, worsening outcomes.* The Commonwealth Fund. https://www.commonwealthfund.org/sites/default/files/2023-02/PDF_Gunja_us_health_global_perspective_2022_exhibits_v2.pdf (accessed June 2, 2025).

Gyawali, B., S. P. Hey, and A. S. Kesselheim. 2019. Assessment of the clinical benefit of cancer drugs receiving accelerated approval. *JAMA Internal Medicine* 179(7):906–913.

Gyawali, B., B. N. Rome, and A. S. Kesselheim. 2021. Regulatory and clinical consequences of negative confirmatory trials of accelerated approval cancer drugs: Retrospective observational study. *BMJ* 374:n1959.

Hemel, D., and L. Ouellette. 2023. Valuing medical innovation. *Stanford Law Review* 75:517–599.

Hopkins, J. S. 2025. Drug development is slowing down after cuts at the FDA. *Wall Street Journal*, April 17. https://www.wsj.com/health/healthcare/drug-development-is-slowing-down-after-cuts-at-the-fda-f22369cf (accessed May 16, 2025).

IHME (Institute for Health Metrics and Evaluation). 2025. *GBD compare.* https://vizhub.healthdata.org/gbd-compare/ (accessed May 16, 2025).

Impact Global Health. 2024. *G-finder.* https://gfinderdata.impactglobalhealth.org/pages/data-visualisations (accessed May 16, 2025).

Karlin-Smith, S. 2024. U.S. FDA's drug center losing shortages, controlled substance leadership with Throckmorton retirement. *Citeline Regulatory*, November 21. https://insights.citeline.com/pink-sheet/agency-leadership/us-fda/us-fdas-drug-center-losing-shortages-controlled-substance-leadership-with-throckmorton-retirement-NOMKUIYP7BDVXEKJ-T66UJFGROI/ (accessed January 15, 2025).

Largent, E. A., A. Peterson, J. Karlawish, and H. F. Lynch. 2022. Aspiring to reasonableness in accelerated approval: Anticipating and avoiding the next aducanumab. *Drugs & Aging* 39(6):389–400.

Lawrence, L. 2024. FDA deputy commissioner Namandjé Bumpus to leave agency. *STAT News*, https://www.statnews.com/2024/12/17/fda-deputy-commissioner-namandje-bumpus-to-leave-agency/ (accessed January 15, 2025).

Lawrence, L., and A. Feuerstein. 2025. Patrizia Cavazzoni, head of FDA's drug center, to leave the agency. *STAT News*, January 10. https://www.statnews.com/2025/01/10/fda-patrizia-cavazzoni-drug-center-head-leaving/ (accessed January 15, 2025).

Lawrence, L., and J. E. Parker. 2025. A running list of senior FDA officials who have left the agency. *STAT News*, April 3. https://www.statnews.com/2025/04/03/fda-senior-officials-exits-departures-list/ (accessed May 16, 2025).

Lemley, M. A., L. L. Ouellette, and R. E. Sachs. 2020. The Medicare innovation subsidy. *New York University Law Review* 95(1):95–96.

McIntyre, C. 2024. Has the FDA lost the plot on surrogate endpoints? *AgencyIQ*, May 28. https://www.agencyiq.com/blog/has-the-fda-lost-the-plot-on-surrogate-endpoints/ (accessed April 3, 2025).

Naci, H., K. R. Smalley, and A. S. Kesselheim. 2017. Characteristics of preapproval and postapproval studies for drugs granted accelerated approval by the U.S. Food and Drug Administration. *JAMA* 318(7):626–636.

NIH (National Institutes of Health). 2024. *Simplified peer review framework.* https://grants.nih.gov/policy-and-compliance/policy-topics/peer-review/simplifying-review/framework (accessed March 14, 2025).

NTEU (National Treasury Employees Union). 2024. *Statement on the Food and Drug Administration and the Commodity Futures Trading Commission.* Statement submitted to the Appropriations Subcommittee on Agriculture and FDA, House of Representatives, April 18. https://www.nteu.org/legislative-action/congressional-testimony/fda-testimony20240823t142315 (accessed April 22, 2025).

Perkmann, M., A. Neely, and K. Walsh. 2011. How should firms evaluate success in university–industry alliances? A performance measurement system. *R&D Management* 41(2):202–216.

Peter G. Peterson Foundation. 2024. *How does the U.S.. healthcare system compare to other countries?* https://www.pgpf.org/article/how-does-the-us-healthcare-system-compare-to-other-countries/ (accessed April 22, 2025).

Phares, S., M. Trusheim, S. K. Emond, and S. D. Pearson. 2024. Managing the challenges of paying for gene therapy: Strategies for market action and policy reform in the United States. *Journal of Comparative Effectiveness Research* 13(12):e240118.

Quandt, K. 2022. The FDA needs to be more flexible in assessing treatments for rare diseases, like the one that seemed to help my son. *STAT News*, September 7. https://www.statnews.com/2022/09/07/the-fda-needs-to-be-more-flexible-in-assessing-treatments-for-rare-diseases-like-the-one-that-seemed-to-help-my-son/ (accessed March 13, 2025).

Sachs, R. E., S. A. Jazowski, K. A. Gavulic, J. M. Donohue, and S. B. Dusetzina. 2022. Medicaid and accelerated approval: Spending on drugs with and without proven clinical benefits. *Journal of Health Politics, Policy, and Law* 47(6):673–690.

Stone, W., and P. Huang. 2025. Some federal health websites restored, others still down, after data purge. *NPR (National Public Radio)*, February 6. https://www.npr.org/sections/shots-health-news/2025/02/06/nx-s1-5288113/cdc-website-health-data-trump (accessed February 6, 2025).

TAGGS (Tracking Accountability in Government Grants Systems). 2024. *Creation of a trusted data broker, development of a data access platform and design of a public private partnership to implement the NIH's Data Counts program for access to quality data.* https://taggs.hhs.gov/Detail/AwardDetail?arg_AwardNum=OT2OD039723&arg_ProgOfficeCode=205 (accessed February 5, 2025).

Wager, E., M. McGough, S. Rakshit, K. Amin, and C. Cox. 2024. *How does health spending in the U.S. compare to other countries?* https://www.healthsystemtracker.org/chart-collection/health-spending-u-s-compare-countries/#GDP%20per%20capita%20and%20health%20consumption%20spending%20per%20capita,%202022%20(U.S.%20dollars,%20PPP-%20adjusted) (accessed April 22. 2025).

Wilkerson, J. 2023. More than 200 FDA staffers have retired in less than a year. *STAT News*, June 6. https://www.statnews.com/2023/06/06/fda-retirements/ (accessed January 15, 2025).

Woodcock, J., K. Berasi, J. Ireland, D. Fox, and T. R. Lal. 2024. October 23. *When exceptions need their own rule: A new rare disease approval pathway.* https://static1.squarespace.com/static/5966cc2220099e91326caaec/t/672241d331b5156a5a7d0f7b/1730298323197/Transcription+Haystack+Project+Panel+10.23.24.pdf (accessed June 2, 2025).

A

Public Meeting Agendas

COMMITTEE ON STRATEGIES TO BETTER ALIGN
INVESTMENTS IN INNOVATIONS FOR THERAPEUTIC
DEVELOPMENT WITH DISEASE BURDEN AND UNMET NEEDS

MARCH 18, 2024

VIRTUAL

CLOSED SESSION

12:00–2:00	Closed Session—Bias and Conflict of Interest Discussion
2:00	Adjourn

APRIL 26, 2024

VIRTUAL

CLOSED SESSION

12:00–2:00   Closed Session—Bias and Conflict of Interest Discussion

OPEN SESSION

2:00–2:05	Welcome Study Sponsors and Introductory Remarks **Ellen MacKenzie** and **Don Berwick,** *Committee Cochairs*
2:05–2:35	Sponsor Presentations Relevant to the Committee's Task **Goutham Kandru,** Gates Ventures **Hannah Menelas,** Peterson Center on Healthcare **Mairin Mancino,** Peterson Center on Healthcare

2:35–3:00   Discussion and Q&A with Sponsors
Ellen MacKenzie and **Don Berwick,** *Committee Cochairs*

CLOSED SESSION

3:00–5:00   Closed Session
5:00   Closing Comments
Ellen MacKenzie and **Don Berwick,** *Committee Cochairs*
Adjourn

JUNE 17, 2024

The Keck Center, 500 Fifth Street, NW
Washington, DC 20001
Room 201

CLOSED SESSION

8:30–7:30   Closed Session

JUNE 18, 2024

The Keck Center, 500 Fifth Street, NW
Washington, DC 20001
Room 206

CLOSED SESSION

8:30–11:00   Closed Session

OPEN SESSION

11:00–12:30   Panel on Decision Making for Therapeutic Innovation
Investment

CLOSED SESSION

12:30–1:00   Closed Session
1:00   Adjourn

JULY 23, 2024

VIRTUAL

CLOSED SESSION

12:00–2:00   Closed Session

OPEN SESSION

2:00–3:10   Guest Speaker: **Peter Kolchinsky,** *Managing Partner and Founder, RA Capital*
             Q&A Session with Committee Members Moderator: **David Scheer,** *Committee Member*
3:10–3:15   Break
3:15–4:25   Guest Speaker: **Aaron Kesselheim,** *Professor of Medicine,* Harvard Medical School; *Faculty Member, Division of Pharmacoepidemiology and Pharmacoeconomics, Department of Medicine,* Brigham and Women's Hospital; *Physician, Phyllis Jen Center for Primary Care,* Brigham and Women's Hospital
             Q & A Session with Committee Members
             Moderator: **Holly Fernandez Lynch,** *Committee Member*
4:25–4:30   Break

CLOSED SESSION

4:30-5:00   Closed Session
5:00   Adjourn

JULY 24, 2024

VIRTUAL

CLOSED SESSION

12:00–2:30   Closed Session

OPEN SESSION

2:30–3:30   Guest Speaker: **Jamie Robinson,** *Professor of Health Economics and Director of the Berkeley Center for Health Technology,* University of California, Berkeley
             Q&A Session with Committee Members Moderator: **Scott Howell,** *Committee Member*
3:30–3:45   Break

CLOSED SESSION

3:45–5:00   Closed Session
5:00   Adjourn

SEPTEMBER 30, 2024

The Keck Center, 500 Fifth Street, NW
Washington, DC 20001
Room 105

CLOSED SESSION

8:30–1:00	Closed Session

OPEN SESSION

1:00	Welcome and Introduction to the Study **Ellen MacKenzie,** *Committee Cochair*
1:05	Presentation **Reshma Ramachandran,** Yale School of Medicine Discussion
1:25	**Inma Hernandez,** *NAM Fellow and Moderator*
2:10	Closing Remarks
2:30–5:15	Closed Session
5:15	Adjourn

OCTOBER 1, 2024

The Keck Center, 500 Fifth Street, NW
Washington, DC 20001
Room 105

CLOSED SESSION

8:30–1:00	Closed Session

OPEN SESSION

1:00–1:05	Welcome and Introduction to the Study **Don Berwick,** *Committee Co-Chair*
1:05–1:25	Presentation **Patrizia Cavazzoni,** Center for Drug Evaluation and Research, U.S. Food and Drug Administration
1:25–1:55	Discussion **Stacey Adam,** *Committee Member and Moderator*
1:55–2:00	Closing Remarks

CLOSED SESSION

2:00–3:00	Closed Session
3:00	Adjourn

NOVEMBER 21, 2024

VIRTUAL

CLOSED SESSION

12:00–1:00   Closed Session

OPEN SESSION

1:00–2:00   Guest Speaker: **Rob Califf,** *Commissioner, Food and Drug Administration*
Q&A Session with Committee Members
Moderator: **Don Berwick,** *Committee Cochair*
2:00–2:15   Break

CLOSED SESSION

2:15–5:00   Closed Session
5:00   Adjourn

NOVEMBER 22, 2024

VIRTUAL

CLOSED SESSION

12:00–2:00   Closed Session

OPEN SESSION

2:00–3:15   Guest Speaker: **Monica Bertagnolli,** *Director, National Institutes of Health*
Q&A Session with Committee Members
Moderator: Ellen MacKenzie, *Committee Cochair*

CLOSED SESSION

3:15–5:00   Closed Session
5:00   Adjourn

DECEMBER 16, 2024

2101 Constitution Avenue
Washington, DC 20418
National Academy of Sciences Members Room

CLOSED SESSION

9:00–1:00   Closed Session

OPEN SESSION

1:00–2:15   Virtual Panel—Patient Engagement in Therapeutic
Development
Pamela Gavin, *Chief Executive Officer, National Organization for Rare Diseases*
Yasmin Ibrahim, *Public Health Program Director, Hepatitis B Foundation*
Marc Boutin, *Global Head of Patient Engagement, Novartis*
Q&A Session with Committee Members
Moderator: Joshua Salomon, Committee Member

CLOSED SESSION

2:15–5:00   Closed Session

DECEMBER 17, 2024

2101 Constitution Avenue
Washington, DC 20418
National Academy of Sciences Members Room

CLOSED SESSION

8:00–1:00   Closed Session

FEBRUARY 3, 2025

The Keck Center, 500 Fifth Street, NW
Washington, DC 20001
Room 105

CLOSED SESSION

9:00–5:00   Closed Session

FEBRUARY 4, 2025

The Keck Center, 500 Fifth Street, NW
Washington, DC 20001
Room 105

CLOSED SESSION

8:30–1:00   Closed Session

B

Committee and Staff Biographical Sketches

Donald M. Berwick, M.D., M.P.P., FRCP, KBE (*Cochair*), is president emeritus and a senior fellow at the Institute for Healthcare Improvement (IHI), an organization he cofounded and led as president and chief executive officer for 19 years. Dr. Berwick is one of the nation's leading authorities on health care quality and improvement. In July 2010, President Obama appointed Dr. Berwick to the position of administrator of the Centers for Medicare & Medicaid Services, a position that he held until December 2011. A pediatrician by background, Dr. Berwick has served as a clinical professor of pediatrics and health care policy at the Harvard Medical School, professor of health policy and management at the Harvard School of Public Health, and as a member of the staffs of Boston's Children's Hospital Medical Center, Massachusetts General Hospital, and the Brigham and Women's Hospital. He has also served as vice chair of the U.S. Preventive Services Task Force, the first "independent member" of the board of trustees of the American Hospital Association, and chair of the National Advisory Council of the Agency for Healthcare Research and Quality. He is a member of the board of directors for Virta Health and NRC Health, on the uncompensated advisory committee for Civica Rx, and formerly on the board of directors for LumiraDx.

He is an elected member of the American Philosophical Society, the American Academy of Arts and Sciences, and the National Academy of Medicine (NAM). Dr. Berwick served two terms on the NAM's governing council, was a member of the NAM's Global Health Board, and currently chairs the NAM Board on Health Care Services. He served on President Clinton's Advisory Commission on Consumer Protection and Quality in the Healthcare Industry. His numerous awards include the 2007 William B. Graham Prize for Health Services Research, the 2006 John M. Eisenberg Patient Safety and Quality Award, and the 2007 Heinz Award for Public Policy. In 2005, he was appointed Honourary Knight Commander of the British Empire by Her Majesty Queen Elizabeth II, the highest honor in the UK for non-UK citizens. He is the author or coauthor of over 200 scientific articles and six books. He received his M.D. from Harvard Medical School and M.P.P. from Harvard Kennedy School.

Ellen MacKenzie, Ph.D., Sc.M. (*Cochair*), is the 11th dean of the Johns Hopkins Bloomberg School of Public Health and a Bloomberg Distinguished Professor. Before becoming dean, Dr. MacKenzie held several leadership positions in the school, most recently as the chair of the School of Public Health's Department of Health Policy and Management. A leading injury prevention and trauma systems expert, Dr. MacKenzie helped shape the field of trauma services and outcomes research. She founded the Major Extremity Trauma Research Consortium, a collaboration of more than 50 U.S. trauma centers and military treatment facilities dedicated to interdisciplinary trials to define best practices for the care of civilian and military trauma patients. Dr. MacKenzie has distinguished herself as an academic leader, always pushing the boundaries of innovative research and the application of that research to programs and policies that make a difference. She sits on the advisory board of the Association of Schools and Programs of Public Health that issues position statements regarding support for increased federal funding across a range of issues in public health.

The Centers for Disease Control and Prevention named Dr. MacKenzie one of 20 leaders and visionaries who have had a transformative effect on the field of violence and injury prevention in the past 20 years. She has also received distinguished career awards from the American Academy of Orthopedic Surgeons, the American Heart Association and the American Stroke Association, the American Trauma Society, and the American Public Health Association (Injury Control Section). In 2018 she was elected a member of the National Academy of Medicine.

Dr. MacKenzie has served on several National Academies of Sciences, Engineering, and Medicine (National Academies) National Research Council committees, most recently on the National Academies Committee on Accelerating Progress in Traumatic Brain Injury Care and Research.

Stacey Adam, Ph.D., is a vice president at the Foundation for the National Institutes of Health (FNIH), leading many public–private partnerships, such as Accelerating COVID-19 Therapeutic Interventions and Vaccines, the Biomarkers Consortium (Cancer and Metabolic Disorders Steering Committees) and their projects, Accelerating Medicines Partnerships–Common

Metabolic Diseases and Heart Failure, Pediatric Medical Devices public–private partnership, Partnership for Accelerating Cancer Therapies, and the Lung Master Protocol clinical trial.

Prior to her time at FNIH, Dr. Adam was a manager at Deloitte Consulting in the federal life sciences and health care strategy practice, where she supported many federal and nonprofit client projects. Before Deloitte, Dr. Adam conducted her postdoctoral fellowship at the Stanford University School of Medicine, where she was both a National Institutes of Health (NIH)– and an American Cancer Society–supported fellow, and she earned her Ph.D. in pharmacology with a certificate in mammalian toxicology from Duke University. She did her B.S. in medical technology/clinical laboratory science from University of Nebraska Medical Center and graduated summa cum laude.

Dr. Adam is a member of the American Association of Cancer Research and the American Society of Clinical Oncology. She received the NIH Directors Award four times between 2020 and 2022 for her work on the partnerships with NIH.

Maria Elena Bottazzi, Ph.D., is the senior associate dean of the National School of Tropical Medicine, the division chief of pediatric tropical medicine, a professor of pediatrics and molecular virology and microbiology, and the codirector of Texas Children's Center for Vaccine Development at Baylor College of Medicine in Houston. She is an internationally recognized tropical and emerging disease vaccinologist, pioneering and leading innovative partnerships for vaccine development to advance a robust infectious and tropical disease vaccine portfolio. Dr. Bottazzi tackles high-burden, neglected, and emerging diseases such as coronavirus, hookworm, schistosomiasis, and Chagas disease, all diseases that disproportionally affect the world's poorest populations.

Dr. Bottazzi is the cocreator of an open-source COVID-19 vaccine technology that led to the development of Corbevax in India and Halal-certified IndoVac in Indonesia. As a global thought leader, she has received national and international highly regarded awards including the 2023 Vilcek-Gold Award for Humanism in Healthcare and the 2023 Holocaust Museum Houston LBJ Moral Courage Award. She was part of the team that received the 2023 David and Beatrix Hamburg Award for Advances in Biomedical Research and Clinical Medicine of the National Academy of Medicine. Dr. Bottazzi was named by *Forbes Latin America* as one of 2022's 100 Most Powerful Women in Central America and as a 2022 Great Immigrant, Great American Honoree of the Carnegie Corporation of New York. In 2022, alongside Dr. Peter Hotez, she was nominated by Texas Congresswoman Lizzie Fletcher for the Nobel Peace Prize. Dr. Bottazzi is a former National Academy of Medicine Emerging Leader in Health and Medicine Scholar.

In 2019 she was member of the ad hoc consensus committee for the report *Stronger Food and Drug Regulatory Systems Abroad*, and in 2021 she was a member of consensus study committee that produced the report *Vaccine Research and Development to Advance Pandemic and Seasonal Influenza Vaccine Preparedness and Response*. She is a member of a technical advisory group for Access to Advanced Health Institute and of the boards of directors for the One Health Research Foundation, Houston Shoulder to Shoulder Foundation, and Consortium of Universities for Global Health.

Dr. Bottazzi obtained her bachelor's degree in microbiology and clinical chemistry from the National Autonomous University of Honduras and a doctorate in molecular immunology and experimental pathology from the University of Florida. Her postdoctoral training in cellular biology was completed at University of Miami and the University of Pennsylvania.

Macarius Mwinisungee Donneyong, M.P.H., Ph.D., is an associate professor at The Ohio State University (OSU) with joint appointments in the colleges of pharmacy and of public health. Prior to joining OSU, Dr. Donneyong was a research specialist at the Division of Pharmacoepidemiology and Pharmacoeconomics at the Brigham and Women's Hospital and Harvard Medical School.

A trained epidemiologist and an expert in pharmacoepidemiology, Dr. Donneyong's background and research interests are in generating real-world evidence of therapeutic products. In particular, he focuses on measuring and understanding how multilevel factors at the individual patient, health care system, and community levels interact to drive racial and ethnic disparities in the use and acceptability of prescribed medications in real-world settings. This line of research has been focused on racial and ethnic disparities in cardiovascular diseases and mental health, especially depression care. Dr. Donneyong is renowned for innovative research that applies data mining techniques to address drug–drug interactions among older patient populations, among whom polypharmacy is the highest. Based on these lines of research, Dr. Donneyong believes that polypills could be the silver bullet to addressing both medication nonadherence and adverse drug–drug interactions caused by polypharmacy.

Dr. Donneyong has been the recipient of several prestigious federal research grants and is a respected figure in the academic community. His expertise has been sought after at various national and international avenues including providing subject matter expertise to policy makers and regulators such as the U.S. Food and Drug Administration (FDA). He is coauthor of the recent FDA report, *External Review of FDA Regulation of Opioid Analgesics*. Dr. Donneyong also serves as a panel member of National Institutes of Health aging, immunology, musculoskeletal and rheumatoid diseases study section and as an ad hoc scientist reviewer for the

Patient-Centered Outcomes Research Institute. Dr. Donneyong is a fellow of both the American College of Epidemiology (ACE) and the International Society of Pharmacoepidemiology. He is a past member of the board of directors of ACE. He received his M.P.H. from Missouri State University and his Ph.D. in epidemiology with a minor in biostatistics from the University of Louisville.

Stacie B. Dusetzina, Ph.D., is a professor of health policy and an Ingram Professor of cancer research at Vanderbilt University School of Medicine, Department of Health Policy. She is a health services researcher focusing on the intersection among health policy, epidemiology, and economics related to prescription drugs. Dr. Dusetzina received her Ph.D. in pharmaceutical sciences from the University of North Carolina at Chapel Hill in 2010 and completed postdoctoral training at the Department of Health Care Policy at Harvard Medical School in 2012. Relevant to the proposed work, prior to graduate training Dr. Dusetzina spent several years working in a contract research organization supporting industry-funded clinical trials, including multiple new drug applications. Her Ph.D. training in pharmaceutical science was obtained from the University of North Carolina Eshelman School of Pharmacy, an academic institution with substantial experience engaging in early-stage discovery and drug development.

Dr. Dusetzina's work has contributed to the evidence base for the role of drug costs and coverage on patient access to care, with a specific focus on access to high-priced drugs and those for rare disease. She has been recognized for her work at a national level, including coauthoring a National Academies of Medicine report, *Making Medicines Affordable*, advising congressional committees and multiple government agencies on prescription drug legislation, and being selected to serve on the Medicare Payment Advisory Commission in 2021. Her work on access to high-priced medications for Medicare beneficiaries was used by the White House and President Biden when promoting and passing the Inflation Reduction Act in 2022. She currently serves as an advisory member for the Institute for Clinical and Economic Review Midwest Comparative Effectiveness Public Advisory Council and on the Medicare Payment Advisory Commission.

Holly Fernandez Lynch, J.D., M.B.E., is an associate professor of medical ethics and law at the University of Pennsylvania. She pursues conceptual and empirical scholarship regarding clinical research ethics and regulation, access to investigational medicines, and Food and Drug Administration pharmaceutical policy, especially approaches to drug development and early access and approval pathways for diseases with unmet treatment needs. She is an expert on priority setting decisions around allocating research resources at the site level, as well as ethical challenges arising in innovative research.

Dr. Fernandez Lynch is a nationally recognized leader at the intersection of bioethics and policy, regularly engaging with patient advocacy organizations, policy makers, and institutional stakeholders. She is a board member of Public Responsibility in Medicine & Research (PRIM&R) and board president-elect of the American Society for Law, Medicine, and Ethics. She was a Greenwall Faculty Scholar from 2019 to 2022, received the inaugural Baruch A. Brody Bioethics Award in 2020, was elected a fellow of the Hastings Center in 2021, and was selected as a National Academy of Medicine Emerging Leader in Health and Medicine in 2022. From 2023 to 2024, she served as a member of the National Academies ad hoc committee Amyotrophic Lateral Sclerosis: Accelerating Treatments and Improving Quality of Life. She is the founder and cochair of the Consortium to Advance Effective Research Ethics Oversight and is a member of the New York University Working Group on Compassionate Use and Preapproval Access.

Dr. Fernandez Lynch has previously worked as an attorney in private practice, representing pharmaceutical clients in regulatory matters. She was also a bioethicist serving in the Human Subject Protection Branch at the National Institutes of Health's Division of AIDS and a senior policy analyst with President Obama's Commission for the Study of Bioethical Issues. From 2012 to 2017 she served as the executive director of Harvard Law School's bioethics and health law research program at the Petrie-Flom Center. She earned graduate degrees in law and bioethics at the University of Pennsylvania.

Howard Scott Howell, M.D., M.B.A., is a health care and life sciences advisor (Blue Line Advisors, LLC), teacher (University of California, Berkeley, and Ohio State University), and cofounder (Synapse Sciences, a U.S.-based biotechnology research association). He began his career as a general internist and became interested in the business and regulation of health care. He returned to school to get an M.B.A. and transitioned into health services administration in academic group practice and then health insurance. Dr. Howell went on to work in the life sciences industries, including at several pharmaceutical companies—GlaxoSmithKline, Jazz Pharmaceuticals, Genentech, and Novartis—retiring as U.S. chief strategy officer of Novartis Pharmaceuticals in May 2022. Dr. Howell joined Novartis in 2017 as vice president and head of U.S. market access, where he was responsible for pricing and contracting, channel management, managed care, hospital systems of care, and patient and specialty services. He also led an initiative at Novartis to employ value-based contracting for medicines, linking pricing and reimbursement rates to specific patient outcomes. He previously consulted for Jazz Pharmaceuticals and FliptRx. He volunteers on the research advisory board of Nationwide Children's Hospital. Dr. Howell has deep expertise in strategic investment and U.S. drug pricing and access; has been teaching, researching, and writing about related topics for many years; and currently cohosts the podcast Prescription for Better Access. Dr. Howell completed his B.S. at the University of Notre Dame, his M.D. at Ohio State University, an internship and residency at Duke University, and an M.B.A. at Duke University.

Mark Olfson, M.D., M.P.H., is the Elizabeth K Dollard Professor of Psychiatry, Medicine, and Law in the Department of Psychiatry at Columbia University Vagelos College of Physicians and Surgeons and a professor of epidemiology at the Columbia University Mailman School of Public Health. He is also a research psychiatrist at New York State Psychiatric Institute. Dr. Olfson's research characterizes national patterns in behavioral health service use, identifies critical gaps between clinical science and practice, and illuminates challenges faced by neglected patient populations including widespread problems in quality of care and inadequate treatment response. Through innovative and influential studies, sensitive to social influences, his research has advanced the understanding of unmet mental health needs and the needs of clinical practice. These studies serve as a foundation for improving treatment access and evaluating the quality, effectiveness, and safety of behavioral health services.

Dr. Olfson graduated from Northwestern University Medical School, completed psychiatric residency training at Yale University, and received a master's in public health at Columbia. He has received numerous awards, including and the Paul Hoch Award from the America Psychopathological Association and the Senior Scholar Health Services Award from the American Psychiatric Association. He has also contributed to National Academy of Medicine reports on preventing mental, emotional, and behavioral disorders in children and youth and on mental disorders and disabilities among low-income children.

Lisa Larrimore Ouellette, Ph.D., J.D., is the Deane F. Johnson Professor of Law at Stanford University Law School as well as a senior fellow at the Stanford Institute for Economic Policy Research. Her research focuses on intellectual property law and innovation policy, including the patenting of publicly funded research under the Bayh-Dole Act. She has applied these ideas to biomedical innovation challenges including the opioid epidemic, the COVID-19 pandemic, and pharmaceutical prices. She has also authored a free casebook, *Patent Law: Cases, Problems, and Materials*, which has been adopted at more than 70 law schools. Prior to her appointment at Stanford Law School, Dr. Ouellette clerked on the U.S. Courts of Appeal for both the Federal Circuit and the Second Circuit. She holds a J.D. from Yale Law School, a Ph.D. in physics from Cornell University, and a B.A. in physics from Swarthmore College.

Edith Adaljisa Perez, M.D., is an internationally recognized translational researcher and cancer specialist and a professor emeritus at the Mayo Clinic. She served as the chief medical officer at Bolt Biotherapeutics from 2020 to 2024. As chief medical officer at Bolt, Dr. Perez oversaw regulatory affairs, pharmacovigilance, biostatistics, and medical affairs for the company's diverse clinical development and early-stage immuno-oncology pipeline. Previously, Dr. Perez was the vice president and head of the bio-oncology medical unit at Genentech, Inc., overseeing all U.S. hematology and oncology medical affairs and, with her team, was involved in leading numerous trials and launching six drugs, including Gazyva, Perjeta, Alecensa, and Tecentriq. Dr. Perez spent the first 20 years of her career at the Mayo Clinic where she was active in teaching, research, and patient care, with a focus in breast cancer and translational biomarkers. She has authored more than 700 peer-reviewed manuscripts and abstracts.

Dr. Perez is on the board of directors for Food Allergy Research Foundation and is a member of the Puerto Rico Science, Technology, and Research Trust; she has been involved in diversity leadership and philanthropic initiatives with the American Society of Clinical Oncology, the American Association for Cancer Research, Stand Up to Cancer, and The DONNA Foundation. She also serves on the editorial boards of multiple academic journals and is a member of the board of directors and the clinical advisory board for Artiva Biotherapeutics.

Dr. Perez earned her M.D. from the University of Puerto Rico School of Medicine in San Juan and completed her residency in internal medicine at the Loma Linda University Medical Center in California. She served as a general internist in the Division of National Health Services Corps in Los Angeles and completed her hematology/oncology fellowship at the University of California, Davis, School of Medicine. Dr. Perez also has pursued leadership, management, and executive development at The Wharton School of the University of Pennsylvania and Harvard Kennedy School in Boston. Dr. Perez is board-certified in internal medicine, medical oncology, and hematology.

Kathryn A. Phillips, Ph.D., is professor of health economics and health services research at the University of California, San Francisco. She founded the UCSF Center for Translational and Policy Research on Precision Medicine (TRANSPERS), which is a global leader in translating new technologies and therapies into clinical care and health policy.

Dr. Phillips's research includes work on how to effectively, efficiently, and equitably implement new technologies and therapies using transdisciplinary approaches and multistakeholder engagement. Dr. Phillips brings expertise in health economics, health policy, therapeutic development, regulatory oversight, and health disparities. She works with industry, venture capital firms, and governmental boards, with a common thread of focusing on how to align investments in research and commercialization with unmet needs. She serves on the evidence review committee with the California Technology Assessment Forum, Institute for Clinical and Economic Review (ICER), and previously chaired the Global Economics and Evaluation of Clinical Genomics Sequencing Working Group (GEECS), which was supported by Illumina Inc. Dr. Phillips previously served on the governing Board of Directors for GenomeCanada and as an advisor to the FDA, CDC, President's Council of Advisors on Science and Technology, and White House Office of Science and Technology, as well as several technology/diagnostic/pharma companies, consulting firms, and venture capital firms. In the past 5 years, she provided consulting advisory services (no longer active roles) to Illumina, Roche, Avia, Association of Community Cancer Centers, and Evidera. She serves as an unpaid volunteer on the Scientific Board of Advisors for Bakar Labs is a life science–focused incubator founded by UC Berkeley and QB3, UC's hub for life science entrepreneurship.

Dr. Phillips is a standing member of the National Academy of Medicine (NAM) Roundtable on Genomic Medicine and Precision Health and has participated in many NAM/National Academies of Sciences, Engineering, and Medicine (National Academies) activities for 25 years, including 11 NAM meetings, most recently as a speaker at the National Academies workshop on "**Opportunities and Challenges for the Development and Adoption of Multicancer Detection Tests**," **and as** a formal speaker at the Roundtable. She has been recognized for her work through lead-authored publications in the highest impact journals that place her in the top 2 percent of authors cited in her field and through service on leading editorial and professional boards, including being named as the founding editor-in-chief of *Health Affairs Scholar: Emerging and Global Health Policy.*

Dr. Phillips earned her B.A. from the University of Texas Austin, M.P.A. from Harvard University, and Ph.D. from the University of California Berkeley. She has been a Visiting Scholar at the Rockefeller Foundation Bellagio Center, Harvard, Memorial Sloan Kettering Cancer Center, London School of Economics, and Brocher Foundation (Switzerland).

Joshua A. Salomon, Ph.D., is a professor of health policy at the Stanford University School of Medicine, senior fellow in the Freeman Spogli Institute for International Studies, and founding director of the Prevention Policy Modeling Lab. Previously, he served as policy analyst at the World Health Organization and as professor of global health at Harvard T.H. Chan School of Public Health.

Trained in health policy and decision science, Dr. Salomon leads multidisciplinary research teams dedicated to producing rigorous, actionable evidence to improve the public's health and reduce health disparities. He has coauthored more than 300 original peer-reviewed research articles and mentored dozens of graduate and postgraduate trainees in health policy, medicine and public health.

His work—supported by the National Institutes of Health, Centers for Disease Control and Prevention, and the Bill & Melinda Gates Foundation—combines data synthesis and mathematical modeling to measure and forecast health outcomes and evaluate public health programs, strategies, and investments. Dr. Salomon has spearheaded methodological innovation in measurement and valuation of population health and disease burden, infectious and chronic disease modeling and forecasting, and cost-effectiveness analysis. His applied modeling work on HIV/AIDS, tuberculosis, viral hepatitis, chronic kidney disease, diabetes, COVID-19, and other major health challenges informs local, state, national, and international policies to improve health and well-being, particularly among underserved populations in the United States and around the world. A major emphasis of his work is on priority setting for health interventions to address unmet population health needs, including assessing the potential health and economic benefits of new and emerging health technologies. Dr. Salomon is a member of the Global Burden of Disease (GBD) Scientific Council, which is responsible for scientific oversight and decision making on study methods.

Dr. Salomon is a member of the Board on Population Health and Public Health Practice at the National Academies of Sciences, Engineering, and Medicine. He received his Ph.D. in health policy and decision sciences from Harvard University.

David I. Scheer, M.S., is a life science entrepreneur, advisor, and company builder with more than 44 years of experience. He is president of Scheer & Company, Inc., a company that provides corporate strategic and transactional advisory services in the life sciences industry. He currently chairs several boards of privately held life science companies, including for Adela, Inc. (an oncology-focused diagnostics company), Refactor Health (a digital health company), and Aprilgen, Inc. (an early-stage pediatric rare disease gene therapy company). Mr. Scheer has previously served in an advisory capacity for many companies as well as for nonprofit research institutions and health care systems involved in research commercialization. He has played a key role as transactionalist, cofounder, and board member/chair for spinoffs from university and corporate research and development. He is currently a cochair of the board of directors for BioCT, member of the Connecticut Bioscience Innovation Advisory Committee, advisor of Wolverine Foundation, and member of the director's advisory committee for the Rutgers Global Health Institute. For a number of years, he was an advisor to the Rett Syndrome Research Trust. He has volunteered as a chair of strategic advisory to the chief executive officer for the National

Organization for Rare Disorders and has moderated numerous panels for their annual Breakthrough Summit. He has also served as organizer and moderator for rare disease and health tech panels at the Yale Innovation Summit and for the Rare Disease Summit at Jackson Laboratories for Genomic Medicine. He has served as a member of the Center for Biomedical Innovation and technology advisory board at Yale University, and he served on a range of initiatives in the public and global health arenas at the Harvard T.H. Chan School of Public Health, including the Harvard Malaria Initiative, the Unfinished Agenda in Infectious Diseases, and an initiative focusing on Cancer in the Developing World with the then-dean, Julio Frenk, and Felicia Knaul. He was a founding member and continues to serve as a member of the New York University Langone Health Compassionate Use and Preapproval Access (CUPA) Working Group.

Mr. Scheer launched his first four companies, all of which saw successful exits, while part of the Health Care Investing Team at Oak Investment Partners. Mr. Scheer was a cofounder of Achillion Pharmaceuticals (acquired by Alexion in 2020, now a unit of AstraZeneca), a publicly held biopharmaceutical company focused on the development and commercialization of small molecule therapeutics for complement-related diseases, and for 21 years he served on its board of directors, including for many years as its chairman of the board. He was also involved in launching, building, and served on the boards of Viropharma (acquired by Shire), OraPharma (acquired by Johnson & Johnson), and Esperion Therapeutics (acquired by Pfizer). He has also launched and served as chair for a variety of other start-ups in the cardiology, neuroscience, ophthalmology, pulmonology, and regenerative medicine arenas. Much of his not-for-profit as well as for-profit activities have been focused on bringing therapies to patients with high unmet needs, including those with rare diseases. He is intricately familiar with the issues that underly successful translation of research into innovation via life science companies. He has given talks at business schools and has moderated and served on a wide range of panels focusing on research commercialization and innovation. Mr. Scheer holds an A.B. degree cum laude in biochemical sciences from Harvard College and an M.S. degree in cellular, molecular, and developmental biology from Yale University.

Wu Zeng, M.D., M.S., Ph.D., is an associate professor at the School of Health at Georgetown University. His research has been centered on health financing, economic evaluation of health interventions (e.g., treatment innovations and technology), and health policy design and evaluation to provide evidence for policy making. He also works on examining health resource flow and allocation to enhance the efficiency of health systems. Dr. Zeng has conducted research in more than 20 countries and has been a senior consultant for many international organizations, including the

World Bank, World Health Organization, the United Nations Children's Fund (UNICEF), the United Nations High Commissioner for Refugees, and the United Nations Population Fund. He is a member of the International Health Economic Association and has served as an advisor to the ministry of health in several countries. Dr. Zeng received his M.D. degree from Fujian Medical University (China) and holds an M.S. degree in global health policy and a Ph.D. degree in social policy from Brandeis University.

NATIONAL ACADEMY OF MEDICINE FELLOWS

Sanket Dhruva, M.D., M.H.S., is the 2023–2025 Greenwall Fellow in Bioethics at the National Academy of Medicine, an assistant professor of medicine at the University of California, San Francisco (UCSF), and a cardiologist at the San Francisco Veterans Affairs Medical Center. His research, clinical, and education interests focus on understanding and strengthening the evidence base for the safe and effective use of drugs and medical devices in diverse populations, with the goal of improving the quality of care and clinical outcomes for patients. He identifies solutions to improve equity in the development and dissemination of these therapies. Dr. Dhruva currently serves on the Medicare Evidence Development & Coverage Advisory Committee and the Institute for Clinical and Economic Review California Technology Assessment Forum. He has authored over 185 peer-reviewed publications and has been funded by the Greenwall Foundation, Department of Veterans Affairs, National Institutes of Health, Food and Drug Administration, National Evaluation System for Health Technology, National Institute for Health Care Management, and Arnold Ventures.

Dr. Dhruva received his B.A. in political science and molecular and cell biology from the University of California, Berkeley. He graduated with an M.D. from UCSF. He completed residency in internal medicine at UCSF and fellowship in cardiovascular medicine at the University of California, Davis. He subsequently completed an M.H.S. at Yale University.

Inmaculada Hernandez, Pharm.D., Ph.D., is a professor at the University of California, San Diego, Skaggs School of Pharmacy and Pharmaceutical Sciences. Dr. Hernandez is a pharmacist and a scholar whose research focuses on improving medication use, outcomes, and equity in access. She has made major contributions to improving transparency in the drug reimbursement system. Dr. Hernandez is a nationally recognized pharmaceutical policy scholar who has made major contributions to improving transparency in the drug pricing and reimbursement system. She was the first to quantify the contribution of innovation versus inflation in the rising trends of drug prices. Dr. Hernandez was recognized on the Forbes 30 under 30 list in

2018, and in 2021 she became the first pharmacist to receive the Academy Health Alice S. Hersh Emerging Leader Award. Dr. Hernandez has pioneered the execution of nationwide person-level geographic information systems analysis to measure inequities in spatial accessibility to the health care infrastructure. This research line commenced in the setting of the COVID-19 pandemic with the development of an app that informed the Pennsylvania Department of Health in the distribution of COVID-19 vaccines to medically underserved areas. Dr. Hernandez has authored over than 100 scientific articles and recently served as the National Academy of Medicine Fellow in Pharmacy.

NATIONAL ACADEMIES STAFF

Alex Helman, Ph.D., is a senior program officer with the Board on Health Sciences Policy at the National Academies of Sciences, Engineering, and Medicine (the National Academies). During her time at the National Academies, Dr. Helman has led numerous activities and consensus studies, including Advancing Clinical Research with Pregnant and Lactating Populations, Improving Representation in Clinical Trials and Research: Building Research Equity for Women and Underrepresented Groups, and Promising Practices to Recruit, Retain, and Advance Women in STEMM Disciplines. She also led the prevention and evaluation working groups for the National Academies' Action Collaborative on Preventing Sexual Harassment in Higher Education. Before joining the National Academies full time, Dr. Helman was as a 2018 Mirzayan Science and Technology Policy Fellow at the National Academies. Prior to her science policy work, Dr. Helman studied vascular contributions to cognitive impairment and dementia in individuals with Down Syndrome. Dr. Helman received her Ph.D. in molecular and cellular biochemistry from the University of Kentucky and her B.S. in biochemistry from Elon University.

Samantha N. Schumm, Ph.D., is a program officer with the Board on Health Sciences Policy at the National Academies of Sciences, Engineering, and Medicine (the National Academies). She is codirector of the study Use of Race and Ethnicity in Biomedical Research. At the National Academies, she has also supported a consensus study, Use of Race, Ethnicity, and Ancestry as Population Descriptors in Genomics Research, as well as planned public workshops and led working groups on topics including workforce development and emerging manufacturing technologies in regenerative medicine. Prior to joining the National Academies in 2021, she studied mild traumatic brain injury at the University of Pennsylvania, using a variety of neuroscience techniques. Dr. Schumm developed a novel computational network model of the hippocampus brain region and analyzed emergent complex behaviors of neuronal networks. Her other interests include writing and promoting effective, inclusive mentorship in the sciences. Dr. Schumm has a Ph.D. in bioengineering from the University of Pennsylvania and a B.S. in biomedical engineering from Yale University.

Andrew March, M.P.H., is a program officer with the Board on Health Sciences Policy of the National Academies of Sciences, Engineering, and Medicine. Most recently, he served as the codirector for the consensus study, *Charting a Path Toward New Treatments for Lyme Infection-Associated Chronic Illnesses.* He has led and contributed to consensus studies on diverse topics in health policy, including clinical research with pregnant and lactating populations, medical product supply chains, and dementia care interventions. Before joining the National Academies in 2018, he conducted research on the intersection of maternal and occupational health at the Center for Research in Occupational Health (CiSAL), and worked in the Department of Clinical Epidemiology and Public Health at the Hospital de la Santa Creu i Sant Pau. Andrew obtained his M.P.H. at the Universitat Pompeu Fabra and his B.S. degree in Biology and Spanish from Roanoke College.

Aja Drain, B.A., is a research associate on the Board of Health Care Services in the Health and Medicine Division at the National Academies of Sciences, Engineering, and Medicine (the National Academies). Prior to her position at the National Academies, she was an award-winning reporter for WAMU/DCist.com and freelanced for National Public Radio (NPR) and Science Friday covering public health and science issues. Before journalism, Ms. Drain conducted research and worked in academic, nonprofit, and industrial organizations throughout her undergraduate career. She has experience in infectious diseases at Washington University School of Medicine, microbiology at Accelerate Diagnostics, HIV/AIDS care at Vivent Health, cancer research at University of Arizona, and diversifying the cancer care workforce at City of Hope. She obtained her B.A. in anthropology: global health and the environment with a minor in biology from Washington University in St. Louis.

Ashley Bologna, M.S., is a research assistant in the Health and Medicine Division at the National Academies of Sciences, Engineering, and Medicine (the National Academies). In addition to this study, she worked on projects initiated by the Committee on Personal Protective Equipment for Workplace Safety and Health. This is a standing committee at the National Academies sponsored by the National Personal Protective Technology Laboratory of the National Institute for Occupational Safety and Health to provide a forum for discussion of scientific and technical issues relevant to the development, certification, deployment, and use of personal protective equipment, standards, and related systems to ensure workplace safety and health. She graduated in 2022 with her master of science in global health at Georgetown University and earned her bachelor of arts in international relations and a bachelor of arts in political science at Virginia Wesleyan University in 2018.

Sharyl J. Nass, Ph.D., serves as the senior director of the Board on Health Care Services and Director of the National Cancer Policy Forum at the National Academies of Sciences, Engineering, and Medicine. To enable the best possible care for all patients, the board undertakes scholarly analysis of the organization, financing, effectiveness, workforce, and delivery of health care, with emphasis on quality, cost, and accessibility. The forum examines policy issues pertaining to the entire continuum of cancer research and care. For more than 2 decades, Dr. Nass has worked on a broad range of health and science policy topics which includes the quality, safety, and equity of health care and clinical trials; developing technologies for precision medicine; and strategies to support clinician well-being. She has a Ph.D. from Georgetown University and undertook postdoctoral training at the Johns Hopkins University School of Medicine as well as a research fellowship at the Max Planck Institute in Germany. She also holds a B.S. and an M.S. from the University of Wisconsin–Madison. She has been the recipient of the Cecil Medal for Excellence in Health Policy Research, a Distinguished Service Award from the National Academies, and the Institute of Medicine staff team achievement award (as team leader).

Clare Stroud, Ph.D., is the senior board director for the Board on Health Sciences Policy at the National Academies of Sciences, Engineering, and Medicine. In this capacity she oversees a program of activities aimed at fostering the basic biomedical and clinical research enterprises; addressing the ethical, legal, and social contexts of scientific and technologic advances related to health; and strengthening the preparedness, resilience, and sustainability of communities. Previously she served as director of the National Academies' Forum on Neuroscience and Nervous System Disorders, which brings together leaders from government, academia, industry, and nonprofit organizations to discuss key challenges and emerging issues in neuroscience research, development of therapies for nervous system disorders, and related ethical and societal issues. She also led consensus studies and contributed to projects on topics such as pain management, medications for opioid use disorder, traumatic brain injury, preventing cognitive decline and dementia, supporting persons living with dementia and their caregivers, the health and well-being of young adults, and disaster preparedness and response. Dr. Stroud first joined the National Academies as a Mirzayan

Science and Technology Policy Graduate Fellow. She has also been an associate at AmericaSpeaks, a nonprofit organization that engaged citizens in decision making on important public policy issues. Dr. Stroud received her Ph.D. from the University of Maryland, College Park, with research focused on the cognitive neuroscience of language, and her bachelor's degree from Queen's University in Canada.

C

Disclosure of Unavoidable Conflicts of Interest

The conflict-of-interest policy of the National Academies of Sciences, Engineering, and Medicine (https://www.nationalacademies.org/about/ institutional-policies-and-procedures/conflict-of-interest-policies-and-procedures) prohibits the appointment of an individual to a committee such as the one that authored this Consensus Study Report if the individual has a conflict of interest that is relevant to the task to be performed. An exception to this prohibition is permitted only if the National Academies determine that the conflict is unavoidable and the conflict is promptly and publicly disclosed.

When the committee that authored this report was established, a determination of whether there was a conflict of interest was made for each committee member, given the individual's circumstances and the task being undertaken by the committee. A determination that an individual has a conflict of interest is not an assessment of that individual's actual behavior or character or ability to act objectively despite the conflicting interest.

Dr. Scott Howell was determined to have a conflict of interest in relation to service on the Committee on Strategies to Better Align Investments in Innovations for Therapeutic Development with Disease Burden and Unmet Needs based on his current role with Blue Line Advisors, LLC, through which he provides ad hoc consulting to companies such as Jazz Pharmaceuticals. He is cofounder of Synapse Sciences, an emerging global drug research network. Dr. Howell owns stock in Novartis and United Health Group.

The National Academies has concluded that for the committee to accomplish the tasks for which it was established, its membership must include at least one person with current expertise and experience in how strategic investments are made by large pharmaceutical companies. As described in his biographical summary, owing to Dr. Howell's experience in market access in the pharmaceutical industry, he understands the strategic investment landscape for commercializing innovative therapeutics to address unmet patient needs and making therapeutics deliverable to patients.

The National Academies has determined that the expertise and experience of Dr. Howell is needed for the committee to accomplish the task for which it has been established. The National Academies could not find another available individual with the equivalent expertise and experience who does not have a conflict of interest. Therefore, the National Academies has concluded that the conflict is unavoidable.

The National Academies believes that Dr. Howell can serve effectively as a member of the committee and that the committee can produce an objective report, taking into account the composition of the committee, the work to be performed, and the procedures to be followed in completing the study.

Dr. Edith Perez was determined to have a conflict of interest in relation to service on the Committee on Strategies to Better Align Investments in Innovations for Therapeutic Development with Disease Burden and Unmet Needs based on her role as chief medical officer at Bolt Biotherapeutics, which develops therapeutics to treat numerous cancers. She is on the board of directors of Artiva Biotherapeutics, an early-stage immunotherapy company, and is a member of the Genentech External Council for Advancing Inclusive Research. Her spouse has stock in Genentech.

The National Academies has concluded that for the committee to accomplish the tasks for which it was established, its membership must include at least one person who has relevant current expertise and experience in all phases of therapeutic development and the biopharmaceutical industry. As described in her biographical summary, owing to her current role as chief medical officer and her past roles as a physician, principal investigator, and vice president and head of bio-oncology at Genentech, Dr. Perez has extensive expertise and experience in basic science research and clinical trials and the biopharmaceutical industry launching novel therapies.

The National Academies has determined that the expertise and experience of Dr. Perez is needed for the committee to accomplish the task for which it has been established. The National Academies could not find another available individual with the equivalent expertise and experience who does not have a conflict of interest. Therefore, the National Academies has concluded that the conflict is unavoidable.

The National Academies believes that Dr. Perez can serve effectively as a member of the committee and that the committee can produce an objective report, taking into account the composition of the committee, the work to be performed, and the procedures to be followed in completing the study. In July 2024, Dr. Perez's role with Bolt Therapeutics changed from chief medical officer to advisor.

Mr. David Scheer was determined to have a conflict of interest in relation to service on the Committee on Strategies to Better Align Investments in Innovations for Therapeutic Development with Disease Burden and Unmet Needs based on his current role as advisor for Nektar Therapeutics and Twist Biosciences. He is a board member of companies advancing novel therapeutics for unmet needs, including OrphAI Therapeutics and BiologicsMD. He is also cochair of BioCT, a nonprofit focused on promoting the growth of the life sciences in Connecticut. The National Academies has concluded that for the committee to accomplish the tasks for which it was established, the committee requires expertise in financial investment, including knowledge about the intricacies of commercialization, investment, and sale of novel therapies. Inherent in this expertise is knowledge about the incentives and regulatory policies that influence innovation and the perceived risks and returns on investment of innovative products. As described in his biographical summary, Mr. Scheer has expertise and experience in financial investment and has deep understanding of the many factors that influence the investment, growth, and sale of companies that translate basic science into novel therapeutics.

The National Academies has determined that the expertise and experience of Mr. Scheer is needed for the committee to accomplish the task for which it has been established. The National Academies could not find another available individual with the equivalent expertise and experience who does not have a conflict of interest. Therefore, the National Academies has concluded that the conflict is unavoidable.

The National Academies believes that Mr. Scheer can serve effectively as a member of the committee and that the committee can produce an objective report, taking into account the composition of the committee, the work to be performed, and the procedures to be followed in completing the study.

In each case, the National Academies determined that the experience and expertise of the individual was needed for the committee to accomplish the task for which it was established. The National Academies could not find another available individual with the equivalent experience and expertise who did not have a conflict of interest. Therefore, the National Academies concluded that the conflict was unavoidable and publicly disclosed it on its website (www.nationalacademies.org).

D

IHME Methods

The Institute for Health Metrics and Evaluation's mapping of drug–use pairs to Global Burden of Disease (GBD) categories involved the following steps: (1) We identified drug uses in the Evaluate Pharma database, covering current drugs for the top 20 pharmaceutical companies, and pipeline drugs for all companies; (2) for validation, we manually mapped drug–use pairs to GBD conditions (causes, risk factors, impairments, injuries, or pathogens) for two companies' current and pipeline portfolios; (3) we then applied a large language model (LLM) to assign drug–use pairs to GBD categories, using the manual mappings as a benchmark for optimizing our input configuration; (4) this highest performing LLM method was used to map the current portfolios of the top 20 pharmaceutical companies and pipeline portfolios for all companies; and (5) we compared these pharmaceutical portfolios by GBD cause to the respective disease burden. The remaining sections in this document provide additional information about each of these steps.

Identification of Drugs and Drug–Use Pairs

We used the Evaluate Pharma database to identify both current pharmaceutical products and pipeline pharmaceutical products. To discover all uses for each of the current drugs, we mapped drug names from the Evaluate Pharma database to reference sources (e.g., Redbook) that specify the use of each drug. For pipeline drugs, we relied on the "specified use" variable in the Evaluate Pharma database.

Manual Mapping of Drug–Use Pairs to Create a Validation Dataset

To assess and optimize the performance of the LLM-based mapping, we created a validation dataset from Pfizer and Sanofi's current and pipeline drug portfolios. Two independent coders mapped each drug–use pair to GBD causes, risk, and injury codes, with a third reviewer resolving any discrepancies. We also compared LLM-based assignments to manual mappings to refine the validation dataset. In addition to causes, other entities were included as options for mapping. The final mapping included 334 causes, 47 injury codes, 18 noncause groupings, 4 risk factors, and the heart failure impairment.

Performance Optimization of an LLM-Based Classification

We supplied the LLM with drug–use pairs and a list of GBD conditions, instructing it to identify the most relevant condition. We refined the prompt to enhance accuracy, using our validation set to evaluate improvements. We also tested different foundational models, including GPT4, o1-mini, and o1-preview. In addition to prompt refinement, we undertook a range of performance optimization approaches. These included the provision of condition keywords generated through a separate LLM process and an adjudication process, whereby we used multiple LLM instances, each with its own medical specialty focus, with a final LLM instance determining the most likely condition assignment.

The table below describes concordance between different LLM approaches that vary according to the foundational model used, whether condition keywords were provided to the LLM, and whether an adjudication

	Level 1 Cause	Level 2 Cause	Level 3 Cause	Level 4 Cause
o1-preview with keywords, adjudicated	98.5%	96.0%	93.9%	92.8%
o1-preview with keywords	98.3%	95.3%	93.0%	93.0%
o1-preview without keywords	97.0%	91.8%	84.8%	83.8%
o1-mini without keywords	97.1%	90.5%	83.5%	85.7%
o1-mini with keywords	97.3%	91.6%	86.5%	91.7%
GPT-4 with keywords	95.3%	87.5%	80.1%	85.6%

process was used. We evaluated concordance at the four levels of the GBD cause hierarchy, with higher levels indicating greater granularity. The highest performing approach was one that uses the o1-preview foundational LLM, condition keywords, and adjudication (limited to instances where the initial classification by the LLM had a confidence level less than or equal to 80 percent).

Application of the Optimized LLM Approach and Postprocessing

Using Evaluate Pharma, we extracted the most recent product data as of February 2025. We then applied our most accurate LLM method for classifying the complete dataset, which includes over 7,000 current and pipeline products from the top 20 companies and over 37,000 additional pipeline products from other companies. Some adjustments were made to the LLM outputs. Specifically, for a small number of cases where the LLM's assignments did not match any valid condition in our hierarchy, we manually mapped the drug–use pairs to the correct condition.

Comparison of Pharmaceutical Portfolios by Cause Against the Corresponding Disease Burden

This analysis encompassed pharmaceutical products globally, both on-market and in development. Comparison of findings to disease burden was made for current drugs to 2021 disease burden and for pipeline drugs to 2030 forecasted disease burden, as defined by GBD 2021.